GLOWING SKIN AND GORGEOUS HAIR

First published in India by HarperCollins *Publishers* 2025
HarperCollins *Publishers* India, Cyber City, Building 10-A,
Gurugram, Haryana-122002, India
www.harpercollins.co.in

2 4 6 8 10 9 7 5 3 1

P-ISBN: 978-93-5489-880-8
E-ISBN: 978-93-5489-961-4

Typeset in 11.5/15.2 Arno Pro
by HarperCollins *Publishers* India Pvt. Ltd

Printed and bound at
Thomson Press (India) Ltd

MIX
Paper | Supporting responsible forestry
FSC® C010615

This book is produced from independently certified FSC® paper to ensure responsible forest management.

HarperCollins *Publishers*, Macken House, 39/40 Mayor Street Upper, Dublin 1, D01 C9W8, Ireland

With blessings of Shree Rajarajeshwari Devi

Disclaimer

The information and content provided in this book are intended for general informational purposes only and should not be considered a substitute for professional medical advice, diagnosis, or treatment. The author and publisher of this book are not medical professionals, and the material presented is not intended to provide medical guidance. Individuals with allergies, sensitivities, or pre-existing medical conditions should exercise caution and consult a qualified medical professional before attempting any of the regimens, practices, or recommendations detailed in this book. Allergies and sensitivities can vary widely from person to person, and what may be safe for one individual might pose risks to another.

The author and publisher disclaim any liability, loss, or risk that may arise directly or indirectly from the use or application of the information contained within this book. Readers are urged to use their own judgment and discretion, in consultation with a qualified medical professional, when considering implementing any of the suggestions, recommendations, or practices described in this book. By reading and using this book, you acknowledge that you have read and understood this disclaimer and agree to use the information presented here responsibly and in consultation with appropriate medical professionals.

CONTENTS

PART 2: THE HAIRCARE GUIDE

PART- 1
THE SKINCARE GUIDE

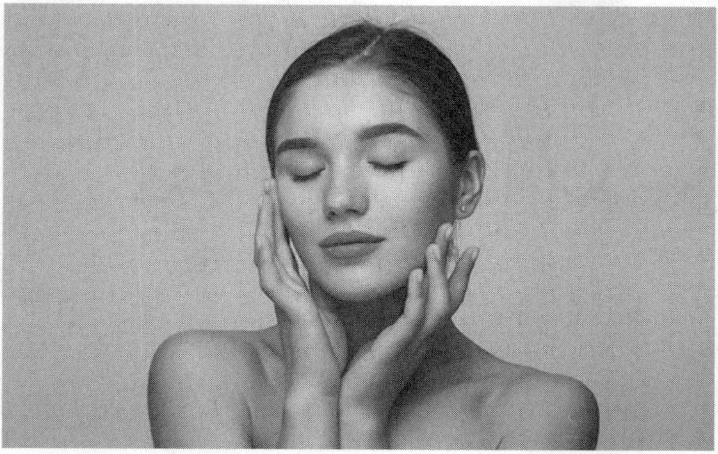

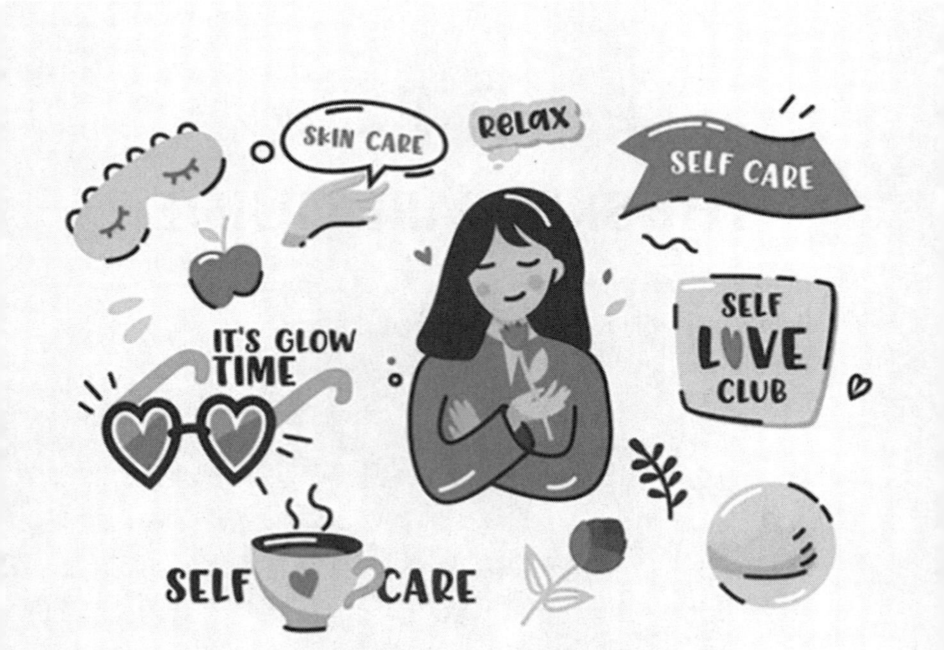
SKIN CARE
RELAX
SELF CARE
IT'S GLOW
TIME
SELF
LOVE
CLUB
SELF
CARE

INTRODUCTION

We all have heard, 'you are what you eat'. Whatever we eat reflects on our skin. Have you ever wondered why some people effortlessly radiate with flawless, glowing skin? The answer lies in the power of their diet and lifestyle choices.

So, why is diet important for a healthy, radiant skin? And how will this book help you in starting a lifestyle that suits you and your skin?

This journey that you're about to embark upon will transform the way you perceive skincare and help you unlock the secrets to a luminous complexion that lasts a lifetime!

We live in a world where makeup has become synonymous with beauty, often masking the true potential of our skin. But deep down, we all yearn for that natural, effortless glow—the kind that makes heads turn and boosts our confidence. It's time to embrace the right habits for healthy, radiant skin, and rediscover the beauty within us.

In this book, we will delve into the importance of diet for achieving a healthy, glowing complexion. We all know that we are what we eat, and this could not be truer in skincare. Every morsel of food we consume manifests on our skin, either enhancing or detracting from its natural beauty.

A glowing, radiant and beautiful skin is the aspiration of many women and men. Countless individuals have embarked on various journeys to achieve these goals, with varying degrees of success. Now it's your turn to take charge and uncover the path to that glowing skin!

In our quest for flawless skin, we often get caught up in external skincare solutions—expensive creams, elaborate treatments and quick fixes. But true skincare begins from within, and it's time to shift our focus back to nurturing our bodies inside out.

Our bodies react differently to stressors, and as we age, the natural processes that keep our skin vibrant and healthy begin to slow down. Merely relying on superficial solutions like SPF-protected moisturizers won't bring out the true beauty of our skin. To attain that coveted natural glow, we must first learn about the power of a balanced diet and a holistic lifestyle.

Maintaining a healthy and skin-friendly diet starts from being mindful of the ingredients in the foods we consume. The secret lies in carefully scrutinizing product labels while shopping. Look out for phrases like 'may contain' or 'made with', as they often indicate potentially harmful ingredients. By making informed choices and avoiding these substances, you can prioritize your skin's health and well-being.

This book serves as your ultimate guide, leading you on a journey to create a nourishing eating plan that promotes a radiant and glowing complexion. You'll discover a handpicked

CHAPTER 1

NORMAL VS AGEING SKIN

What happens to your skin as you grow older? How does your skin support nutrition as you age?

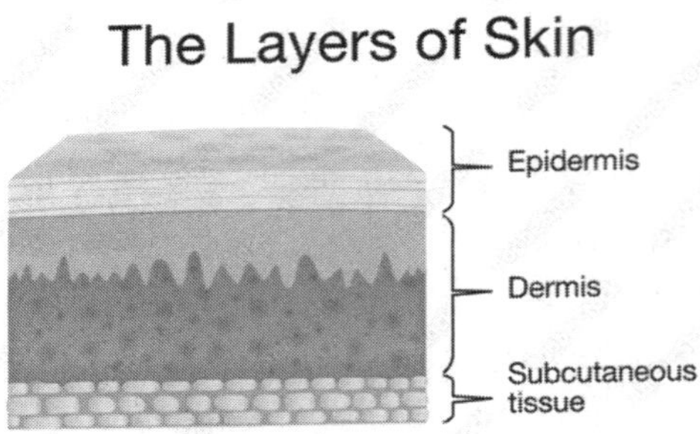

The **skin** is the largest organ of the body. It protects us from germs and injury, as well as regulates temperature and plays a role in excretion. The skin is made up of three layers: epidermis, dermis and hypodermis.

The **epidermis** is the outermost layer of skin. It is made up of dead cells that continually shed as new ones take their place. The epidermis protects us from germs, bacteria and ultraviolet rays by producing melanin (pigment) that absorbs ultraviolet light.

The **dermis** is situated below the epidermis. It contains collagen fibres (which give strength), elastic fibres (which give resiliency), nerve endings, sweat glands (which produce sweat), sebaceous glands (which produce oil), hair follicles (from which hair grows) and blood vessels.

The **hypodermis** is also known as subcutaneous tissue because it's beneath your actual skin tissue. It consists mainly of fat cells that store energy for later use in times of need. It also produces collagen fibres to support your body's weight when you stand on your feet all day long or carry heavy objects around without feeling sore afterwards.

YOUNGER SKIN vs. AGING SKIN

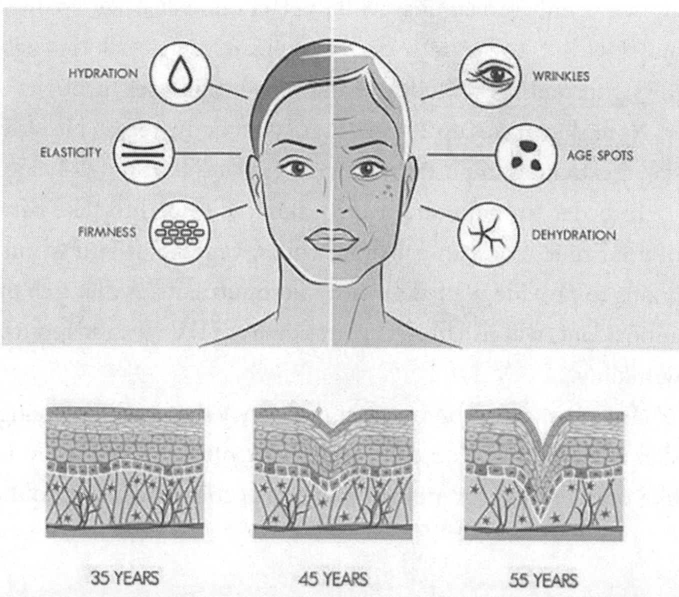

Skin ageing is a universal phenomenon that touches every individual, regardless of age, gender or cultural background. It is a subject of great interest and concern, as our skin is not only a visible reflection of our inner health and vitality but also a significant aspect of our identity and self-image.

One of the most important aspect of your beauty routine is your skincare. There are many skin types, depending on a person's race and lifestyle habits. Your face is like a project you want to start working on sooner than later. So if you want to save money and time, you need to know the difference between young and ageing skin.

Skin changes with age, but it doesn't have to be a depressing process. One of the first signs of ageing is that the skin loses its elasticity, and no matter how much you pull or tug, you won't get your skin back to what it used to be. But with age comes wisdom, and there are ways to combat skin ageing.

We're only too familiar with the fact that as we age, so does our skin. But how exactly does this occur? Let's walk through the significant age-affecting changes your skin goes through.

Your skin makes up 20 per cent of your body weight. Healthy skin is extremely important for our overall health and well-being.

In order to maintain healthy skin, you need to take care of your diet. You can eat more fruits, vegetables and whole grains to provide your skin with micronutrients. A diet rich in antioxidants will also protect your skin from UV rays and reduce wrinkling.

The most common nutrient deficiency that leads to ageing skin is vitamin C. You can get enough vitamin C from foods like orange juice, grapefruit juice, broccoli, brussels sprouts and strawberries. But if you're not eating enough fruits and vegetables daily, then it might be beneficial for you to take supplements of this vitamin.

WRINKLES

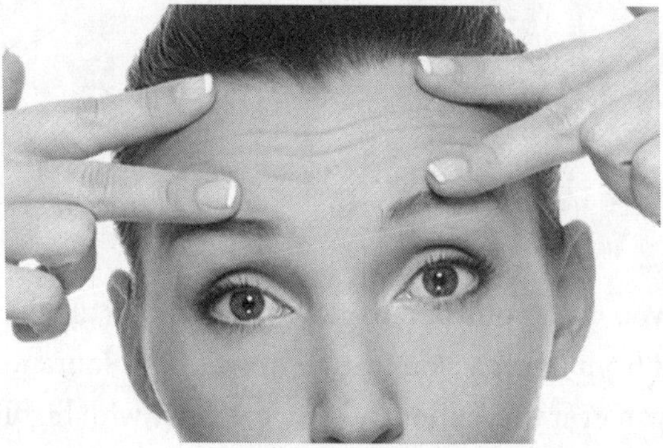

What exactly are wrinkles? Wrinkles, like skin tone and texture, are determined by the amount of hydration your skin has. This can be affected by factors like climate, diet and lifestyle.

As people get older, it's one of the most common skincare concerns they have. Fine lines and creases in the skin are frequently caused by sun damage. Other factors, such as facial expressions or genetics, can also contribute to them.

The first step is to understand what causes wrinkles in the first place. Wrinkles are caused by collagen loss, the protein that gives your skin its elasticity and strength. Collagen is a protein that makes up the connective tissue in our skin and other tissues in our body. When we lose collagen, our skin looks wrinkled and loose.

UNEVEN TEXTURE

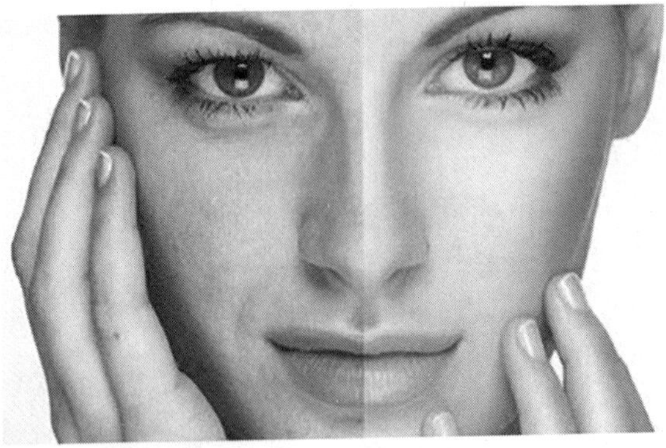

Do you want your skin to glow evenly? Well, if you've ever suffered from uneven skin texture or skin discolouration, then before you ever think about adding products with highlighting properties to your skincare routine or makeup, ensure that you understand why these things occur in the first place. It's a fact that most ethnicities are prone to uneven skin texturing and pigmentation. The reason is an increase in melanin production in the epidermis layer of the skin (which is a natural process). As a result, dark spots and hyperpigmentation occur.

Nutrition is important to maintain an even skin tone and texture. A healthy diet rich in fruits, vegetables, whole grains and lean protein will keep you young and healthy.

SAGGING SKIN

I'm sure you've seen it before. You look in the mirror and notice sagging skin or fine lines, especially around your mouth

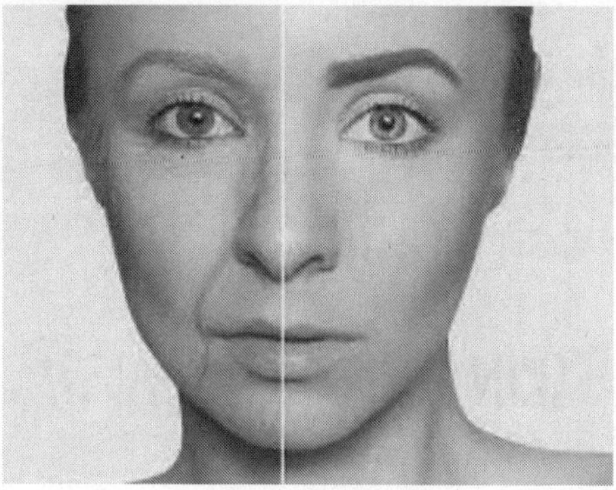

and eyes. But did you know that our skin is literally one of our organ systems! Yes, that's true!

It's the organ of touch, the protection system and sensory organ. When we look at people who are older, we can see their skin lacks elasticity and tissue strength, which leads to sagging effects.

A combination of factors can contribute to sagging skin, but one of the most common culprits is poor nutrition. If you're not getting enough protein, vitamins and minerals in your diet, your body will start breaking down its own tissue for fuel—which is a recipe for sagging skin.

Myth: Sagging skin is a sign of ageing.

Fact: Sagging skin means your body is not effectively producing collagen as it should. This can be due to the process of ageing or a diet with little to no collagen sources.

CHAPTER 2

SKIN AND GUT HEALTH

Did you know that the gut is the unsung hero of our body? It's not just an ordinary organ system; it's an incredible powerhouse that keeps us healthy and vibrant! Picture this: trillions of bacteria, both good and bad, coexist in your gut, working tirelessly to aid digestion, produce essential vitamins and defend against harmful invaders.

Imagine your gut as a bustling city, with its main residents being these tiny superheroes called probiotics. They are the good bacteria that keep everything in balance and ensure the smooth functioning of your gut. Without them, our digestive system would be in chaos, leading to discomfort and various health issues.

But here's where it gets even more fascinating: Remember those childhood days when it seemed like your skin had magical powers to heal? Whether it was a scraped knee or a little bump, our parents would clean the wound, kiss it, and voilà! It would miraculously disappear. However, the real secret behind this amazing healing ability lies in probiotics.

Our skin, the largest organ in our body, is a true multitasker. It shields us from germs, regulates temperatures and even stores fat. But its superhero power is acting as a formidable barrier against toxins in our environment. Guess who supports our skin's defence system? You guessed it: probiotics!

Probiotics not only work wonders within our gut but also play a vital role in maintaining healthy and resilient skin. They work their magic by enhancing the skin's protective barrier, preventing harmful substances from penetrating and causing damage. With a strong barrier, our skin can ward off toxins, pollutants, and other environmental nasties, keeping it clear, radiant, and healthy.

So, probiotics work silently but effectively to maintain the balance, health, and well-being of our gut and skin. By supporting digestion, boosting immunity, and safeguarding against harmful substances, they play an essential role in keeping us thriving.

Now, the next time you think about the incredible powers of your gut and skin, remember the tiny but mighty probiotics working their magic behind the scenes. So, let's give a shout-out to these incredible superheroes and make sure we nourish them with a healthy diet and lifestyle choices.

Your skin and gut health go hand in hand. If your skin is not healthy, it won't be able to do its job as well as it should. This might make you wonder why the gut and skin are interconnected.

The relationship between gut and skin is truly fascinating and goes beyond what meets the eye. Your gut, often referred to as your second brain, plays a crucial role in absorbing nutrients from the foods you eat and converting them into energy. But its influence doesn't stop there—it also has a profound impact on the health and appearance of your skin.

Surprisingly, many people are unaware of the significant impact that gut health has on their skin. Your gut health affects not only your digestion but also your overall well-being, including your mood, immune system and hormone regulation. It's a vital component of your body's metabolism, influencing processes like nutrient absorption, toxin elimination and even the balance between fat and muscle mass.

According to Byrd, Belkaid, and Segre (2018), the human skin microbiome plays a crucial role in skin health.

Did you know that the same beneficial bacteria that reside in your gut can also be found on your skin?

These bacteria play a crucial role in maintaining a healthy balance by breaking down food into essential nutrients and fending off harmful bacteria that can trigger skin issues like acne or eczema.

So, the next time you reach for that sugary snack or opt for a nutrient-dense meal, remember that you're not just feeding your body—you're nourishing your gut and nurturing your skin. Strive for a diet that supports a diverse and balanced gut microbiome, and watch as your skin reflects the vibrant health that lies within.

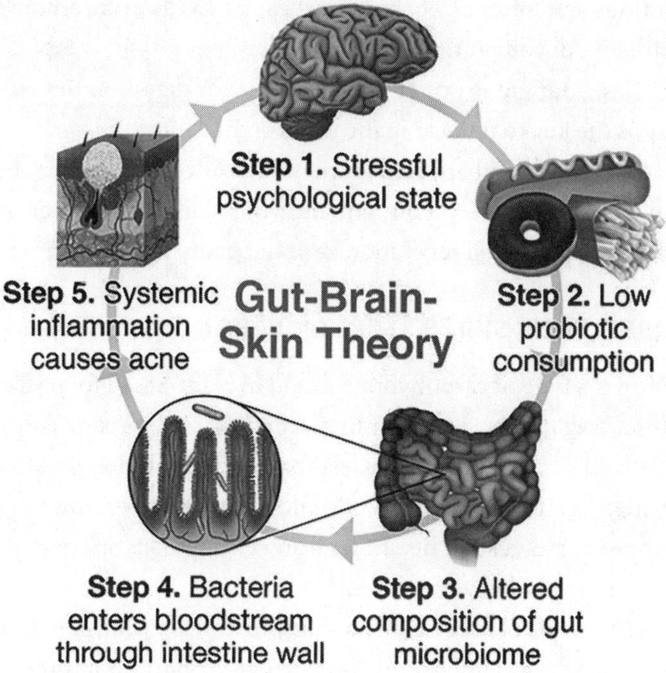

What you eat affects your skin more than you may realize; in fact, 80 per cent of your immune system resides within your gut.

WHY IS GUT HEALTH IMPORTANT FOR SKIN?

Imagine a world where your skin radiates a natural, lit-from-within glow, where breakouts and blemishes become distant memories, and your complexion is as vibrant as a summer sunset. Achieving this dreamy skin is not about slathering on potions and lotions but about nurturing a hidden powerhouse within you: your gut.

Yes, your gut is not only responsible for digestion but also holds the key to unlocking the true potential of your skin.

It's time to embark on a journey of discovery, exploring the relationship between your gut and your skin and uncovering the secrets that will revolutionize your beauty routine forever.

FIBRE: YOUR SKIN'S SECRET WEAPON

Fibre is a type of carbohydrate found in plant-based foods like fruits, vegetables, whole grains, legumes, and nuts. It is not digested by the body but instead passes through the digestive system relatively intact. While fibre is primarily known for promoting digestive health and preventing constipation, its benefits extend beyond the gut.

The magic of fibre lies in its ability to nourish your skin from the inside out. Here's how fibre can contribute to improved skin health:

1. **Healthy Gut**: At its core, fibre plays a pivotal role in promoting a healthy gut microbiome. Your gut is home to trillions of bacteria, both beneficial and harmful. By acting as a prebiotic, fibre serves as nourishment for the good bacteria in your gut. This nourishment encourages a balanced and diverse microbial environment, leading to reduced inflammation and enhanced overall skin health. So, by simply incorporating fibre-rich foods into your diet, you're cultivating an environment that fosters radiant skin from within.

2. **Detoxifies Skin**: Fibre also supports your skin's detoxification process, ensuring that toxins and impurities are efficiently eliminated from your body. By promoting regular bowel movements, fibre keeps your digestive system running smoothly, preventing the build up of harmful substances that can trigger skin issues like acne and breakouts. Embracing fibre as part of your skincare routine means giving your skin the clean slate it needs to thrive, resulting in a clearer and healthier complexion.
3. **Better Nutrient Absorption:** Fibre is a champion when it comes to enhancing nutrient absorption. Your skin craves essential vitamins, minerals, and antioxidants for optimal health, and fibre helps ensure that these nutrients are effectively absorbed from the foods you eat. By improving nutrient assimilation, fibre equips your skin with the building blocks it needs for cell regeneration, collagen production, and overall vitality. So, by adding fibre-rich foods to your plate, you're not only nourishing your body but also unlocking the true potential of your skin.
4. **Blood Sugar Balance:** High blood sugar can contribute to skin concerns such as acne and premature ageing. Fortunately, fibre-rich foods come to the rescue by helping regulate blood sugar levels. Unlike refined carbohydrates that cause rapid spikes, fibre slows down digestion and the release of sugar into the bloodstream. This steady release of sugar helps prevent skin inflammation and breakouts, empowering you to achieve a calmer and more radiant complexion.

PROBIOTICS: NATURE'S BEAUTY POTION

Our skin is home to a vast array of microorganisms that play a crucial role in maintaining our overall health. Among these microorganisms are probiotics, tiny organisms that can work wonders for our skin by providing essential nutrients and even combating common skin problems.

Probiotics are a type of microorganism that naturally reside in our digestive system, both in humans and other animals. Their presence is vital for maintaining a healthy balance in our gut, which is crucial for our overall well-being. But here's the exciting part: they also contribute to the health of our skin! Probiotics help reduce inflammation, which can improve the appearance of ageing signs and acne scarring, leaving your skin looking more youthful and refreshed.

Incorporating probiotics into your diet is an essential component of promoting both gut and skin health. You can find probiotics in various foods, such as yoghurt, pickles, and sauerkraut. By including these probiotic-rich foods in your daily meals, you're providing your skin with the nourishment it needs to thrive.

If you're looking for an addition to your diet that can help with your skin problems, you might want to consider trying probiotics for skin health.

WHY PROBIOTICS FOR SKIN

1. **Balances the skin's natural bacteria:** Probiotics help maintain a healthy balance of bacteria on the skin, keeping harmful bacteria in check and supporting a more harmonious environment for your skin.

2. **Strengthens the skin's protective barrier:** Probiotics aid in strengthening the skin's natural barrier, which acts as a shield against external factors like pollution and irritants, helping to prevent damage and sensitivity.
3. **Reduces skin inflammation:** Probiotics have anti-inflammatory properties that soothe redness and calm inflammation, which can be beneficial for conditions like acne, rosacea, and sensitive skin.
4. **Supports skin healing:** Probiotics assist in the healing process of the skin by promoting cell regeneration and tissue repair, helping wounds, scars, and other skin concerns.
5. **Soothes and calms irritated skin:** Probiotics have a calming effect on the skin, reducing discomfort and irritation caused by various factors like dryness, allergies, or environmental aggressors.
6. **Promotes a healthy and vibrant complexion:** By improving overall skin health, probiotics contribute to a more radiant and youthful appearance, enhancing the natural beauty of your skin.

PREBIOTICS

Imagine prebiotics as the nutrient-rich soil for your skin's garden to flourish. Like a gardener tending to their plants, prebiotics provide a nourishing feast for the beneficial bacteria (probiotics) residing on your skin, just like fragrant petals enticing bees. By giving these tiny microbial allies the sustenance they crave, prebiotics create a vibrant ecosystem on your skin's surface, fostering a harmonious balance that exudes health and vitality.

In the ancient land of India, where the bond between humans and nature is revered, prebiotics and your skin form a harmonious partnership. Acting as an Ayurvedic guru, prebiotics guide your skin on a transformative journey, strengthening its protective barrier, soothing inflammation, and revealing a luminous complexion. This journey invites you to embrace the wisdom of centuries-old traditions, uncovering the secret to true radiance.

WHY PREBIOTICS FOR SKIN

1. **Nourishes the skin's good bacteria:** Prebiotics act as a source of nutrition for the beneficial bacteria on your skin, helping them thrive and maintain their population, which in turn supports a healthier skin environment.
2. **Maintains a healthy pH balance:** Prebiotics assist in maintaining the skin's natural pH balance, which is important for the optimal functioning of the skin's protective barrier and the prevention of harmful bacteria growth.
3. **Enhances skin hydration:** Prebiotics improve the skin's ability to retain moisture, keeping it well-hydrated, plump, and supple, which is essential for a healthy and youthful complexion.
4. **Boosts the skin's immune system**: By fostering the growth of beneficial bacteria, prebiotics strengthen the

skin's immune defences, aiding in the protection against infections, environmental stressors, and other threats.

5. **Improves nutrient absorption:** Prebiotics enhance the skin's capacity to absorb and utilize essential nutrients from skincare products or a balanced diet, ensuring that your skin receives the necessary nourishment for its vitality and appearance.

Food Sources of Probiotics and Prebiotics

Probiotics	Prebiotics
• Tempeh • Kombucha • Kefir • Yoghourt • Buttermilk • Curd • Cottage cheese(paneer) • Kimchi • Miso	• Chicory root • Garlic • Onions • Bananas • Barley • Oats • Apples • Cocoa • Flaxseeds

Myth: If your parents have wrinkles, you will have them too.
Fact: Low antioxidant intake can cause early wrinkles, whether your ancestors had them or not.

CHAPTER 3

SKIN: THE MIRROR OF OVERALL WELL-BEING

Beyond its aesthetic appeal, your skin acts as a vital interface between your body and the external world. It plays a crucial role in protecting you from harmful elements, regulating body temperature, and even providing important sensory experiences. But did you know that your skin's health is intricately connected to your overall health and wellness? It's true! The condition of your skin can be a telltale sign of what's happening inside your body. So, let's embark on a journey to discover why nurturing your skin is not only about beauty but also about safeguarding your overall health and vitality. Get ready to uncover the secrets that lie beneath the surface as we delve into the fascinating connection between your skin and your well-being.

Skin contains sweat glands, hair follicles, oil glands, and nerve endings. Sweat glands are responsible for producing sweat, which cools our bodies when we sweat.

- Hair follicles produce hair and help protect against bacteria that can cause infections in wounds or cuts.
- Oil glands produce sebum, an oily substance that helps keep skin soft and moist.
- Nerve endings in the skin send signals to the brain about touch, pain, pressure and temperature changes in our environment, so we can respond accordingly.

Skin is also important because it's a visual indicator of our overall health status. If someone has a rash or a burn on their skin, we might assume that it's an indication that something else is wrong with their body, such as an infection or inflammation.

HORMONAL HEALTH

The food we choose to consume has a direct influence on our hormonal health, as it provides the essential building blocks for hormone production and activity within the body. Every bite we take acts as a nutritional cue that sets off a cascade of reactions, affecting the delicate balance of hormones that regulate various bodily processes.

Hormonal balance plays a crucial role in maintaining healthy skin, and the food we eat can influence hormone levels, which in turn can impact skin health.

Hormonal imbalance is one of the most common reasons for skin issues. Hormones can affect the way your body functions and the way you look. When you are young, your hormones are in balance, but as you age, they start to change. This is normal, but sometimes it can lead to problems like acne breakouts or a change in the texture of your skin. Skin is affected by hormones because they transport nutrients, oxygen, and other things through your blood to reach every cell in your body.

I know, I know. It's not just your hormones, that's for sure. But I wanted to start with this because it's so important.

You may have noticed that you've gained weight since your teenage years. You may be wondering if this is due to a hormonal imbalance. Hormonal balance is essential for a healthy body, and when it goes awry, so does your metabolism.

What causes hormonal imbalance? There are many factors that could lead to this condition, but the most common ones include:

- **Processed foods:** Consuming a diet high in processed foods, such as fast food, packaged snacks and sugary beverages, can disrupt hormonal balance. These foods are often lacking in essential nutrients and can contribute to inflammation in the body, leading to skin problems like acne, dullness and uneven texture.
- **Excessive sugar intake:** Consuming too much sugar can cause a spike in blood sugar levels, leading to an increase in insulin production. This can disrupt hormone regulation and contribute to hormonal imbalances that negatively impact the skin. Excess sugar consumption is often associated with skin issues like acne, premature ageing and inflammation.
- **Insufficient nutrient intake:** A diet lacking in essential nutrients, such as vitamins, minerals and antioxidants, can contribute to hormonal imbalances and affect skin health. Nutrients play a vital role in maintaining hormonal

balance and supporting the overall function of the skin. Inadequate intake of these nutrients can result in skin problems like dryness, dullness and a compromised complexion.

KIDNEY PROBLEMS

The kidneys produce hormones that regulate blood pressure, red blood cell production and bone density. Kidneys also remove waste products from the body through urine. If they aren't working properly, waste products can build up in your system and cause problems with your health—including your skin.

Kidney failure can cause dry or itchy skin, as well as hair loss, rashes, and a dull complexion.

It's not uncommon for people with kidney problems to experience other skin conditions, too. For instance, some people with kidney disease experience a condition called pruritus (itchy skin). This is sometimes caused by changes in the body's electrolyte balance and can be treated with over-the-counter creams and lotions.

Many people don't realize that drinking two litres (about 64 ounces) of water each day can help your kidneys filter out waste. You also need to eat foods high in potassium, such as bananas or avocados, because they help flush out extra sodium in your body. If you're taking medications for high blood pressure or heart disease, you might want to skip the salt shaker when eating at home.

If you have kidney problems, you're more likely to get infections in your skin, such as fungal infections or boils.

OBESITY

Obesity can affect the skin in a number of ways. It can lead to stretch marks and cellulite, but it also increases the risk of skin cancer and other conditions. The extra weight that comes with obesity puts additional pressure on the skin, causing it to stretch out and form stretch marks.

The dimples of your skin—cellulite

Cellulite is another common symptom of obesity. Cellulite occurs when fat cells push against the tissue below the surface of your skin, causing a dimpling effect. Because cellulite is caused by fat deposits rather than excess water, it cannot be removed by diet or exercise alone; however, losing weight may reduce its appearance somewhat by helping you drop some pounds.

HYPER/HYPOTHYROIDISM

The thyroid gland produces two hormones that regulate metabolism: triiodothyronine (T3) and thyroxine (T4). The former speeds up the body's metabolic rate; the latter slows it down. When your thyroid isn't working properly, these hormones can get out of balance, causing an array of symptoms that can affect your complexion in many ways.

Thyroid issues often cause skin problems, including dryness, flaking, and a dull complexion.

The thyroid hormone controls the function of almost every organ in the body, including the skin. When your thyroid gland is underactive (hypothyroidism), you may have dry skin with fine wrinkles and a loss of elasticity. You may also experience hair loss and brittle nails. When your thyroid is overactive (hyperthyroidism), you may have oily skin with acne or an oily scalp and hair loss from pulling out your hair as it grows.

LIVER

It is one of the organs similar to your skin. Because the work they do in our bodies is very similar. Both of them are involved in avoiding the entry of harmful bacteria and toxins.

Poor liver function has been linked to a variety of skin conditions, including acne, eczema, and psoriasis. Dry, itchy skin, acne, and a dull complexion can all be symptoms of a tired, overworked liver.

Your liver processes everything you eat, drink, and consume, so it's critical to keep it as healthy as possible.

Skin health is affected by many factors, including diet, exercise and stress levels. The most important factor is nutrition: what you eat affects your skin directly and indirectly through its effect on your body weight and metabolism.

Myth: Poor skin health only affects the appearance of the skin.

Fact: Skin health can have broader implications beyond appearance. Skin conditions like eczema, psoriasis and dermatitis can cause discomfort, itching and pain, and even affect a person's quality of life. Additionally, some skin conditions may indicate underlying systemic health issues that require medical attention.

CHAPTER 4

WHY IS MENTAL HEALTH IMPORTANT FOR YOUR SKIN?

When we feel happy and energized, it often shows in the appearance of our skin. A healthy mental state can contribute to a radiant and glowing complexion, reflecting our inner vitality and confidence. On the other hand, when we're experiencing mental distress or emotional strain, it can manifest as dull, dry and tired-looking skin.

Nutrition plays a crucial role in supporting both mental and skin health. A balanced and nutrient-rich diet can provide the essential vitamins, minerals and antioxidants that our bodies need to function optimally. B vitamins, such as thiamine (vitamin B1) and riboflavin (vitamin B2), are particularly important for brain health and maintaining a positive mood.

In times of mental health challenges, it's not uncommon for our bodies to become depleted of vital nutrients. Therefore, paying attention to nutrition for mental health becomes crucial. By consuming foods that are rich in essential nutrients, we can support our mental well-being while also nourishing our skin.

Here's how your mental health is connected to your skin:

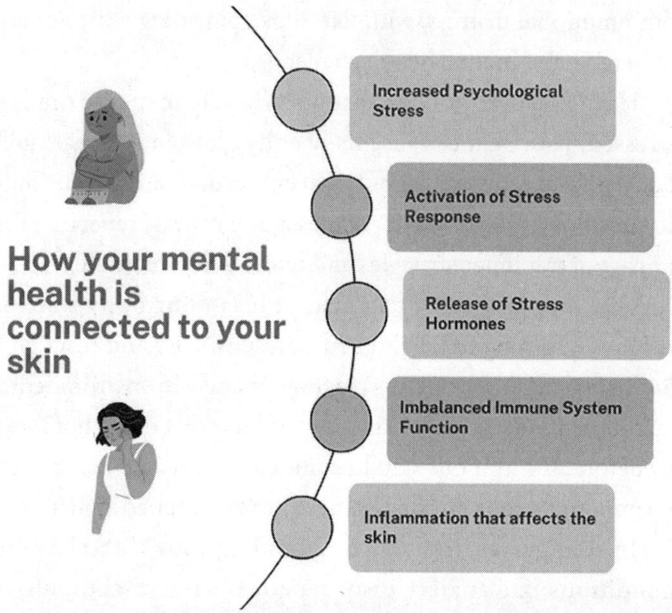

WHAT DOES YOUR SKIN SAY ABOUT YOUR MENTAL HEALTH?

Our skin serves as a fascinating window into our mental well-being. While it's important to remember that everyone's experiences are unique, our skin can provide valuable insights into our emotional state. Let's explore some ways in which our skin reflects our mental health, but remember, these signs may vary from person to person.

When stress, anxiety or depression take hold, they can unleash a cascade of systemic inflammation that affects our skin. This inflammation can aggravate common skin conditions such as acne, eczema, psoriasis, and rosacea. It's as if our skin mirrors our emotional distress, with flare-ups coinciding with periods of heightened mental health challenges.

Have you ever noticed that when you're mentally tired or stressed, your skin can lose its healthy glow and appear dull? Lack of sleep, stress, and emotional exhaustion can all contribute to this. It is as if our skin becomes a dull canvas, reflecting the impact of our inner struggles and making us look tired.

Our mental health can also unleash our body's stress response, leading to heightened skin sensitivity and reactivity. Suddenly, we find ourselves reacting strongly to environmental factors, irritants, or even skincare products that never bothered us before. It's as if our skin becomes an emotional barometer, responding to our internal battles with heightened vigilance.

In some cases, individuals grappling with mental health conditions like anxiety disorders or obsessive-compulsive disorder (OCD) may engage in skin-picking or hair-pulling behaviours. These repetitive actions not only inflict physical damage but also leave scars and hair loss in their wake. It's a visible manifestation of the emotional turmoil they face.

While these insights are valuable, it's crucial to remember that they're not definitive indicators of one's mental state. Mental health is deeply personal and multifaceted, and seeking professional support is vital. However, by paying attention to our skin and recognizing potential correlations with our mental well-being, we can adopt a more holistic approach to self-care. This involves addressing both our external appearance and internal emotional health, paving the way for a more vibrant and balanced life.

Remember, taking care of our mental health is a journey, and small steps towards self-care and seeking support can make a world of difference.

THE DYNAMIC DUO: OMEGA-3s AND B-COMPLEX VITAMINS FOR SKIN AND MENTAL HEALTH

Omega-3 Fatty Acids

Omega-3 fatty acids are a type of essential fat that is crucial for both your mental health and your skin's vitality. These fats, primarily found in fatty fish like salmon, mackerel, and sardines, as well as walnuts and flaxseeds, offer a multitude of benefits.

When it comes to your mental well-being, omega-3s have been shown to play a significant role. Studies have linked higher intakes of omega-3 fatty acids with a reduced risk of depression and improved mood. They are involved in the production of neurotransmitters like serotonin, which regulates mood and emotions.

But that's not all—omega-3s also work wonders for your skin. These fatty acids possess anti-inflammatory properties, helping to calm redness, reduce skin sensitivity, and alleviate conditions such as acne and eczema. Omega-3s are essential for maintaining the integrity of the skin's barrier function, keeping it hydrated and protected against environmental stressors.

B-Complex Vitamins

B-complex vitamins are essential for both your mental health and your skin's health. They play a crucial role in supporting brain function and regulating your mood. When you don't get enough of these vitamins, it can lead to symptoms of depression, anxiety, and problems with memory and focus. That's why it's important to make sure you're getting an adequate intake of B-complex vitamins to support your mental well-being and improve cognitive performance.

But B-vitamins don't just benefit your mind; they are also great for your skin! They help promote the turnover of skin cells, which keeps your complexion healthy and vibrant. B vitamins, like biotin and niacin, are especially good for your skin, hair, and nails. They can improve the appearance of your skin by enhancing its texture and reducing dryness or redness.

Here are some tips on how to get the most out of B-complex vitamins:

1. **Fortified plant-based milk:**

- Look for unsweetened varieties of almond milk, soy milk or coconut milk that are fortified with B vitamins.
- Use fortified plant-based milk as a base for smoothies, cereal, or in your coffee or tea to increase your B vitamin intake.

2. **Leafy green vegetables:**

- Incorporate a variety of leafy greens into your salads, stir-fries, or smoothies.

- Opt for darker greens like spinach and kale, which tend to have higher B vitamin content.
- Consider lightly steaming or sautéing your greens to maximize nutrient absorption.

3. **Legumes and lentils:**

- Include legumes like beans, lentils and chickpeas in your meals.
- Make soups, stews or chilli with legumes as a protein-rich and B vitamin-packed alternative.
- Experiment with different recipes like bean salads or lentil curries to keep your meals interesting.

4. **Fortified gluten-free products**:

- Check the labels of gluten-free bread, cereals and pasta for B vitamin fortification.
- Look for products that specifically mention B vitamin content or enrichment.
- Use fortified gluten-free products as a convenient and easy way to boost your B vitamin intake.

5. **Nuts and seeds:**

- Snack on a handful of almonds, walnuts or pumpkin seeds for a nutrient-rich snack.
- Sprinkle ground flaxseeds or chia seeds on your smoothies, yoghurt or oatmeal for an added B vitamin boost.

6. **Gluten-free whole grains:**

- Replace gluten-containing grains with gluten-free alternatives like quinoa, brown rice, millet or buckwheat.

- Cook these grains as a side dish or use them as a base for salads or grain bowls to incorporate them into your meals.

7. **Nutritional yeast:**

- Use nutritional yeast as a dairy-free and gluten-free cheese substitute.
- Sprinkle nutritional yeast on popcorn, roasted vegetables or pasta dishes for a savoury, cheesy flavour and a B vitamin boost.

Myth: Clear skin equates to good mental health.
Fact: While having clear skin can boost confidence, it doesn't necessarily indicate good mental health. Mental health is multifaceted and influenced by various factors beyond physical appearance.

CHAPTER 5

COMPONENTS FOR HEALTHY SKIN

We all know that healthy skin is the holy grail we're all after. It's that radiant, glowing complexion that makes you feel like a million bucks and gives you an extra spring in your step. Now, take a look around—the skincare market is bursting at the seams with products that promise miraculous results. They dazzle us with fancy packaging and slick marketing, but here's the truth: the real skin-boosting components can be found right in your food!

Yes, you read it right. Your kitchen holds the key to long-lasting and budget-friendly skin health.

Let's uncover the delicious secret to unlocking your skin's true potential!

1. Marine Collagen

Collagen is the most abundant protein in the human body. It gives structure to our skin, bones, tendons, cartilage and muscles.

Amino acids are the building blocks of protein, which is why marine collagen contains high levels of amino acids like glycine, proline and hydroxyproline. These amino acids are known to be effective in improving the appearance of wrinkles, fine lines and age spots on the skin.

But you're probably wondering why marine collagen? Because it is the best source for collagen available!

Marine collagen contains an amino acid called hydroxyproline that helps strengthen the proteins in your skin. The more collagen you have, the healthier your skin will be. It is a great way to improve the appearance of the skin, whether it is in a bottle or a food supplement. Despite being used for centuries, only recently has marine collagen been found to contain all the amino acids that are needed in our bodies. Isn't that fascinating?

Take the quiz below to know if you really require Nutracy Lifestyle's Marine Collagen.

1. Are you older than 26 years of age?

   ☐ Yes

   ☐ No

2. Are you experiencing a noticeable decline in skin elasticity or firmness?

   ☐ Yes

   ☐ No

3. Do you have fine lines or wrinkles that you would like to reduce the appearance of?

   ☐ Yes

   ☐ No

4. Is your skin prone to dryness or lack of hydration?

☐ Yes

☐ No

5. Have you noticed a decrease in skin smoothness or texture?

   ☐ Yes

   ☐ No

6. Are you looking to support your skin's overall health and healing processes?

   ☐ Yes

   ☐ No

If you answered YES to all of the above questions, you need to try my very own beauty collagen powder.

Here's how the purest collagen will be beneficial for you:

- **Skin hydration:** Collagen helps retain moisture in the skin, leading to improved hydration and a more supple appearance.
- **Wrinkle reduction:** Some studies suggest that collagen supplementation may help reduce the appearance of fine lines and wrinkles, improving overall skin texture.
- **Elasticity and firmness:** Marine collagen is believed to support the production of new collagen fibres, which can help improve skin elasticity and firmness.

- **Skin health and healing:** Collagen is an essential component in wound healing and may help promote the healing process of damaged or injured skin.

How to get marine collagen in your diet:

1. Include in your meals three to four servings of fish and shellfish in a week.
2. Include vitamin C and zinc-rich foods every day.
3. Use bone broth in gravies.
4. Choose a good marine collagen supplement (or a collagen booster supplement if vegetarian).

2. Retinol

Retinol is a form of vitamin A that works by unclogging pores and removing dead skin cells, promoting cell turnover, increasing cell turnover and collagen production, reducing hyperpigmentation (dark spots), and improving elasticity.

Here's why you need retinol in your diet:

1. Research has shown that retinoids are effective in treating acne as well as other skin issues such as wrinkles, roughness and age spots.
2. This ingredient is also known to improve fine lines and wrinkles by strengthening the fibrous connective tissue in the dermis layer of the epidermis.
3. Additionally, retinoids improve tone by stimulating collagen production in the deeper layers of the skin, which helps reduce pigmentation issues.

4. Retinol is one of the most powerful antioxidants available, so it can help reverse damage caused by free radicals in the body.

Include the following in your diet to make it retinol-rich.

Plant Products	Animal Products
• Carrots	• Tuna
• Papaya	• Salmon
• Spinach	• Beef liver
• Bell peppers	• Egg yolk
• Sweet potatoes	• A2 cow's milk
• Pumpkin	• Ghee
• Apricots	
• Lettuce	
• Butternut squash	
• Cantaloupe	

3. Hyaluronic Acid

Hyaluronic acid is best known for its ability to reduce the appearance of fine lines and wrinkles by removing built-up dead cells from the skin's surface. This can improve the overall appearance of the complexion, help prevent further signs of ageing and even reduce the appearance of acne scars.

Hyaluronic acid helps improve overall skin tone by reducing the appearance of redness and discolouration caused by sun exposure, acne or other conditions that affect the complexion. It also improves skin texture by making it smoother and more youthful-looking.

A good diet is the foundation for great-looking skin. The right foods will give your skin a healthy glow and a beautiful, radiant look.

Where can you get Hyaluronic acid? It's in your food!

- Almonds and cashews
- Green leafy vegetables
- Bone broths
- Cucumber
- Apple with skin
- Banana
- Lemon

4. Vitamin C

Around 70 per cent of Indians are deficient in vitamin C. If you are one of them, you might need to take extra care of your skin.

Vitamin C is an antioxidant that promotes collagen production and helps reduce the appearance of fine lines and wrinkles. It also helps boost the skin's natural glow, giving it a healthy, youthful appearance.

While you might have come across many serums loaded with vitamin C, our traditional foods are not behind.

Your daily vitamin C checklist: Tick the ones you consumed yesterday.

- ☐ Amla
- ☐ Guava
- ☐ Oranges
- ☐ Kiwi
- ☐ Bell peppers
- ☐ Strawberries
- ☐ Papaya
- ☐ Tomatoes
- ☐ Lemon
- ☐ Broccoli
- ☐ Pineapple
- ☐ Mangos
- ☐ Cantaloupes

Myth: Vegan/Vegetarian collagen exists.
Truth: Real collagen is only marine collagen. The products you see in the market as vegetarian collagen have nutrients that can help make body collagen but do not have it directly.

CHAPTER 6

TRIGGERS FOR BAD SKIN HEALTH

Our skin contains blood vessels, nerves, lymphatic vessels and sweat glands. Together, these structures produce millions of different chemicals that trigger different responses in the body.

It's incredible how the food we put into our bodies can either be a secret weapon for flawless skin or an accomplice in our skin struggles. By gaining a deeper understanding of how our food choices impact our skin, we can make smarter decisions that lead to a radiant and healthy complexion.

Your skin is your body's first line of defence against the outside world. It protects you from bacteria, viruses, and other potentially harmful substances that could enter through open wounds or cuts in the surface.

KNOW WHAT'S CAUSING OUR SKIN ISSUES

Trigger 1: Vitamin Deficiency

You know, we all talk about how vitamins are essential for our overall health, but did you know they also play a major role in the health of our skin? It's true! When we don't get enough of certain vitamins, our skin can start acting up and showing some serious symptoms. It is like a cry for help from our body, telling us to pay attention to our nutrient intake.

Let's start with **vitamin A**. If we're lacking in this superhero nutrient, our skin can become dry, rough, and scaly. It's like a desert out there! To add to the trouble, vitamin A deficiency can even mess with our vision, causing night blindness. Talk about a double whammy!

Now, let's talk about the **B vitamins**. When we don't get enough of **vitamin B1 (thiamine)**, our skin can become dry and scaly, and our eyes might turn all red and irritated. It's like a bad case of dry skin and angry eyes all rolled into one.

Vitamin B2 (riboflavin) deficiency is no joke either. It can lead to changes in hair colour, making it go all wonky on us. That's not all! Our skin can become fragile and easily damaged; our appetite might disappear; and we might even experience some mental confusion. Talk about a rollercoaster ride!

Oh, and let's not forget about **vitamin B3 (niacin)**. When we don't get enough of this vitamin, our hair might start to thin out, our joints might ache, and our muscles can become weak. It's like a whole army of symptoms marching in, making themselves known.

Last but not least, we have **vitamin C**. You know, the one that's often associated with oranges and all things citrusy. Well, if we don't get enough of it, our lips can become dry and cracked, like we've been wandering in a desert for days. And get this—our hands and feet might develop these little red dots that turn into painful cracks when exposed to the air. Ouch!

So, next time you're slacking on your vitamin intake, remember that it's not just your overall health at stake but also the health of your skin. Give your body the nutrients it needs, and your skin will thank you with a healthy, radiant glow.

Trigger 2: Dairy

Ah, dairy, the beloved delight for many. But did you know that dairy might have a not-so-delightful connection to our skin issues? Brace yourself, because it's time to uncover the potential dark side of dairy when it comes to our skin.

The theory goes that milk and dairy products can be troublemakers when it comes to acne and other blemishes. How, you ask? It all boils down to inflammation and clogged pores. Milk has been found to increase sebum production, that oily substance that can make our skin feel like it's staging a rebellion. When sebum and bacteria join forces on our skin's surface, they can create a party zone for inflammation. We're talking about the release of a trouble-causing substance called prostaglandin E2 (PGE2), which can pave the way for acne to rear its unwelcome head.

Wait, there's more! Dairy contains hormones that can disrupt the natural balance of our skin's glands and, you guessed it, cause acne. Those hormones are sneaky troublemakers that aren't supposed to be there in the first place. You see, most commercially available dairy products come from cows that are given antibiotics to keep them healthy, as they tend to fall ill due to overstimulation of their reproductive organs. These hormones can find their way to us, wreaking havoc and triggering skin problems like acne and even rosacea.

Speaking of rosacea, dairy may not be a friend to those dealing with this condition. Rosacea is known for causing redness and inflammation in the cheeks and nose. It is a pesky situation brought about by an overproduction of skin cells and the creation of blood vessels beneath the skin's surface. Now, dairy foods like milk, yoghurt, cream cheese, and butter contain a protein called casein, which is naturally found in cow's milk. This little protein can be a trigger for those with rosacea, causing those blood vessels to dilate and become inflamed when faced with environmental factors like sun exposure or stress.

So, if you're dealing with acne or rosacea, it might be worth considering a break from dairy. Give your skin a chance to breathe without those potential hormone disruptors and irritating proteins. Explore dairy-free alternatives and see if your skin responds with a happier, clearer complexion. It's all about finding what works best for you and your skin's unique needs.

Trigger 3: Refined Sugar

Sugar, although a staple in many diets and a popular ingredient in numerous food products, can be a significant trigger for skin issues. The effect of sugar on the skin goes beyond its impact on blood sugar levels.

Here's an expanded explanation of how sugar can affect the skin and why it's important to be mindful of its consumption:

- **Glycation and Advanced Glycation End Products (AGEs):**

Excessive sugar consumption can contribute to a process called glycation, where sugar molecules bind to proteins in the body, forming harmful molecules known as advanced glycation end products (AGEs). AGEs can damage collagen and elastin, the proteins responsible for maintaining the skin's structure and elasticity. When collagen and elastin fibres are compromised, the skin becomes less supple, leading to the formation of wrinkles, sagging, and overall premature ageing.

- **Inflammation:**

Consuming high amounts of refined sugar and sugary treats can cause a rapid spike in blood sugar levels. This spike triggers the release of insulin, a hormone that helps regulate blood sugar. However, elevated insulin levels can also lead to increased inflammation throughout the body, including the skin. Inflammation can manifest as redness, swelling, and a higher likelihood of developing acne breakouts and other skin conditions.

- **Acne:**

Sugar consumption, particularly foods with a high glycemic index (such as sugary snacks, white bread, and soda), can potentially contribute to the development or exacerbation of acne. High-glycemic foods cause a rapid increase in blood sugar levels, which prompts the release of insulin and insulin-like growth factor 1 (IGF-1). These hormones can stimulate sebum production and trigger an inflammatory response in the skin, leading to clogged pores and acne breakouts.

- **Collagen Degradation:**

Sugar intake can also impact collagen quality and contribute to its degradation. The excess sugar in the bloodstream can lead to a process called cross-linking, where sugar molecules attach themselves to collagen fibres, making them stiff and less functional. This compromised collagen structure can result in a loss of skin elasticity and firmness, contributing to the formation of fine lines and wrinkles.

To maintain healthier skin, it's essential to watch our sugar intake and opt for natural alternatives or low-glycemic sweeteners when possible. Choosing fresh fruits, which contain natural sugars along with beneficial vitamins and antioxidants, can be a better option for satisfying our sweet cravings. Additionally, maintaining a well-balanced diet that includes plenty of fruits, vegetables, whole grains, and lean proteins can provide the necessary nutrients for skin health.

Trigger 4: High Glycaemic Food

Let's dive into the world of high glycaemic index (GI) foods and their impact on our skin. Brace yourself for some eye-opening insights into how these foods can potentially wreak havoc on our skin's health.

What exactly are high-GI foods? They're the speed racers of the food world, causing our blood sugar levels to skyrocket in no time. When we consume these quick-release carbohydrates, our blood sugar goes on a wild ride, leading to a surge in insulin production. Now, here's where things get tricky for our skin.

Insulin, the hormone responsible for regulating blood sugar, also has a not-so-pleasant side effect on our sebaceous glands. It can signal these oil-producing glands to go into overdrive, pumping out more oil than our skin really needs. As we all know, excess oil can be an invitation for clogged pores and unwelcome breakouts.

There's more! High-GI foods also have a knack for triggering inflammation in our bodies, and inflammation and happy skin are not exactly best buddies. When our blood sugar levels go haywire, it sets off a chain reaction that releases inflammatory substances. This inflammation can manifest on our skin as redness, irritation and even flare-ups of conditions like acne or eczema.

Now, let's talk about those high-GI culprits that we should watch out for. We're talking about those sugary goodies that make our taste buds sing—think fluffy white bread, decadent cakes, tempting cookies, and those oh-so-sweet sugary drinks. They may give us a momentary rush, but they can leave us dealing with the aftermath.

But fear not, my friend! We have a solution to keep our skin smiling and our blood sugar levels in check. It's all about embracing the world of low-GI alternatives. Think wholesome whole grains, nourishing legumes, refreshing fruits and colourful veggies. These champions of the plate provide a slower release of energy, keeping our blood sugar levels stable and our skin happy.

Here are some low glycemic index foods you can have:

Food	Glycemic Index (GI)
Lentils (moong dal)	25
Chickpeas (chana)	33
Kidney beans (rajma)	27

Food	Glycemic Index (GI)
Black-eyed peas (lobia)	38
Split peas (toor dal)	35
Barley (jau or jowar)	25
Brown rice	50
Whole wheat roti	45
Oats	55
Quinoa	53
Sweet potatoes	54
Tomatoes	15
Cucumbers	15
Mushrooms	10
Almonds	5

Trigger 5: Artificial Sweeteners

Alright, let's talk about those tricky artificial sweeteners and how they can mess with our skin. Get ready for some eye-opening information that might make you rethink your sugar-free cravings.

The American Journal of Clinical Nutrition has been digging into artificial sweeteners since way back in 1973, when they hit the market. Guess what? They've found some not-so-sweet stuff. These sweeteners could potentially mess with our glucose metabolism and insulin sensitivity. Yikes!

But here's the juicy part: These sneaky artificial sweeteners have also been linked to skin issues like acne. How exactly they do that is still a bit of a mystery, but it seems like they can throw our body's systems out of whack, and our skin pays the price.

Now, here's another shocker. Artificial sweeteners may also play games with our weight. Believe it or not, some studies suggest that folks who use these sweeteners may end up gaining weight, even when they don't eat more calories or slack on exercise. How does that happen? Well, it's like these sweeteners mess with our sugar cravings, making us want more of the real stuff. This can lead to over-indulging and packing on the pounds.

But hey, not everyone reacts the same way. Some people might be more sensitive to these sweeteners, and they could experience annoying side effects like headaches or bloating. Others might not notice a thing. We're all unique, right?

So be cautious with those artificial sweeteners. Sure, they promise fewer calories, but their potential impact on your skin and overall well-being shouldn't be taken lightly. Instead, why not opt for natural sweeteners like honey, maple syrup, or even good old fruit? They might be a wiser choice in the long run.

Trigger 6: Gluten

Gluten is a protein found in wheat, rye and barley. It's used to make dough for bread and other baked goods. Gluten is also often used in processed foods like breads, cakes and pastas. This makes it difficult for people who have celiac disease or non-celiac gluten sensitivity (NCGS) to avoid gluten if they eat packaged foods like these.

Gluten can cause skin issues for many people because it's a protein that can cause inflammation in the body. The inflammation caused by gluten may make your skin look or feel itchy or red—especially on your face.

The inflammation caused by gluten is caused by an immune response to proteins called protamine (specifically glutenin), which are present in the grain. This protamine contains two types of glutamate, one of which is known as glutamic acid. Glutamate has been shown to trigger an immune response that causes inflammation throughout the body.

There is limited evidence of increased inflammation or irritation on the skin, but it's possible that gluten may be related to other inflammatory issues. For example, studies suggest that people with acne have higher levels of intestinal permeability, a condition that occurs when the lining of the intestine becomes damaged, allowing some substances to leak into the bloodstream.

Gluten has also been linked to heightened production of cortisol, a hormone involved in stress responses and metabolism. Cortisol can cause inflammation on the skin as well as promote fat storage around the belly area.

Trigger 7: Whey Protein

Let's dive into the world of whey protein, a popular ingredient found in many skincare products. You know what's pretty fascinating? Whey protein is actually a by-product of cheesemaking. Who would've guessed that something cheese-related could do wonders for your skin?

Here's the lowdown: Whey protein is a powerhouse of protein goodness, which we all know is essential for our bodies.

Not only does it aid in muscle recovery after intense workouts, but it also has some impressive abilities to repair damaged skin tissue. It's like a superhero for your skin, swooping in to save the day!

But wait, there's a twist in this tale. Some studies suggest that consuming whey powder or protein powder may have a downside: acne. Yep, that frustrating skin problem that can pop up for anyone, regardless of gender. However, it's important to note that these studies aren't entirely conclusive. They simply indicate a common trend.

Interestingly enough, reducing the consumption of whey protein powder seems to improve skin conditions for many people. It's like giving acne a run for its money! Of course, everyone's skin is unique, and what works for one person may not work for another. But hey, if you're dealing with those pesky breakouts, why not give reducing your whey protein powder intake a shot? It might just be the game-changer your skin needs.

Remember, though, that there's no one-size-fits-all solution. Experimentation is key, and what matters most is finding what works best for you and your fabulous skin. So go ahead, keep exploring, and embrace your natural beauty—you've got this!

Trigger 8: Ultra Processed foods

When it comes to satisfying our taste buds, there's no denying the allure of processed and fried foods. From that crispy bag of chips to the convenient fast food meals, these guilty pleasures often find their way into our diets. However, while they may provide immediate gratification for our taste buds, they might not be doing our skin any favours.

Processed and fried foods have gained popularity for their convenience and addictive flavours. Unfortunately, these foods are typically loaded with unhealthy fats, artificial additives, and high levels of sodium. These culprits can wreak havoc on our body's natural balance and have a profound impact on the health and appearance of our skin.

Here's how these will affect your skin:

- One of the key concerns with processed and fried foods is their **unhealthy fat content**. These foods are often prepared using trans and saturated fats, which can increase inflammation in the body. Inflammation is a well-known trigger for various skin conditions, including acne, eczema and psoriasis. The excessive consumption of these unhealthy fats can disrupt the delicate balance of our skin, leading to breakouts, redness and even accelerated signs of ageing.
- In addition to unhealthy fats, processed and fried foods also contain **artificial additives**. These additives are used to enhance flavour, prolong shelf life, and improve texture. However, they can have detrimental effects on our skin. Some additives, such as artificial food colouring and flavourings, have been linked to allergic reactions and skin sensitivities in certain individuals. Furthermore, excessive consumption of these additives can put an additional burden on our body's detoxification systems, potentially leading to an accumulation of toxins that may manifest as skin issues.

- High levels of sodium are another common characteristic of processed and fried foods. Sodium is a necessary nutrient in our diet, but excessive intake can lead to water retention and bloating. These effects can make our skin appear puffy and dull, detracting from its natural radiance. Moreover, the high sodium content can dehydrate our skin, leaving it dry and prone to irritation.

While it's unrealistic to completely eliminate processed and fried foods from our lives, it's important to be mindful of their impact on our skin. Opting for fresh, whole foods as much as possible can provide our skin with the nourishment it needs to stay healthy and vibrant. Incorporating a variety of fruits, vegetables, lean proteins and whole grains into our diet can supply our body with essential vitamins, minerals and antioxidants that support skin health.

Moreover, making small changes to our cooking methods can have a significant impact. Instead of frying foods, consider alternative cooking techniques like baking, grilling, or steaming. These methods retain more of the natural nutrients in our ingredients while minimizing the formation of harmful compounds that can affect our skin.

Trigger 9: Excessive Iodine Consumption

Iodine is a vital mineral that plays a crucial role in maintaining our overall health. It can be found in various foods, such as seaweed, seafood and iodized salt. However, it's important to note that for some individuals, consuming excessive amounts of iodine-rich foods may trigger acne breakouts. The reason behind this lies in the potential of high iodine levels to stimulate oil production in the skin, leading to clogged pores and unsightly blemishes. Therefore, striking a balance in your iodine intake becomes essential in order to keep your skin calm and clear.

When it comes to our health, finding the right equilibrium is often the key, and iodine is no exception. While it is an essential mineral required for the proper functioning of our thyroid gland, excessive intake can sometimes result in unintended consequences for our skin. Acne breakouts caused by high iodine levels can be particularly frustrating, especially for those who are prone to acne or have sensitive skin.

Here are four reasons why you need to be mindful of excessive consumption of iodine:

- **Increased sebum production:** Iodine has the ability to stimulate the production of sebum, the natural oil that keeps our skin lubricated. While sebum is necessary for maintaining healthy skin, an excess amount can clog pores and lead to acne. The overproduction of sebum caused by high iodine levels creates an environment where pores are more likely to become congested, resulting in the formation of pimples, blackheads and whiteheads.
- **Clogged pores:** When sebum production is accelerated due to excess iodine, it can mix with dead skin cells, bacteria, and other impurities on the surface of the skin. This combination can block the pores, preventing them from properly releasing sebum and impurities. As a result, the pores become clogged, leading to the development of acne lesions and potentially exacerbating existing acne.

- **Inflammation:** Clogged pores can trigger inflammation within the skin. When the pores are blocked, the accumulated sebum and impurities create an ideal environment for bacteria to thrive, leading to an inflammatory response. The body's immune system reacts to the presence of bacteria, resulting in redness, swelling, and the formation of painful acne lesions.
- **Hormonal imbalance:** Excessive iodine consumption can disrupt the delicate balance of hormones in the body. The thyroid gland, which plays a crucial role in regulating hormone production, relies on iodine to function properly. However, an excess of iodine can interfere with thyroid function and potentially disrupt the balance of other hormones, including those that regulate sebum production and skin health. Hormonal imbalances can contribute to acne development and exacerbation.

Interesting Fact

Seaweed, a common ingredient in many Asian cuisines, is often lauded for its high iodine content. While it offers various health benefits, including being a great source of minerals and antioxidants, excessive seaweed consumption may contribute to acne breakouts. Similarly, seafood, particularly fish and shellfish, can also be rich in iodine. While seafood is generally considered a healthy part of a balanced diet, it's advisable to monitor your intake, especially if you notice a correlation between high seafood consumption and acne flare-ups.

Maintaining a healthy and balanced diet is vital for our overall well-being. When it comes to iodine, this means being aware of the potential effects it can have on our skin and taking proactive steps to find the right balance. If you suspect that high iodine intake may be contributing to your acne breakouts, it can be helpful to consult a dermatologist or a healthcare professional. They can provide personalized advice and recommend suitable dietary modifications to address your specific concerns.

CHAPTER 7

IT'S IN YOUR GENES

Skin types are a big topic for many, but it's also important to talk about genetics as one factor that can affect skin. Genetics is the underlying cause of your skin type, but it's not the only thing you need to consider. Let's go through each skin type and figure out where genetics fit into your life.

SKIN TYPE AND GENETICS

The genes that determine your skin type are porphyria cutanea tarda (PC), lactase persistence (LP), and apolipoprotein E 4/4 (APOE). The first two genes determine how much pigment you produce. The APOE gene determines how fast you lose pigment as you age.

Skin type is determined by the combination of these genes. If you inherit two copies of the PC gene, you will have normal skin; if you inherit one copy, you will have strongly pigmented skin; and if you inherit none, you will have very lightly pigmented skin.

Skin Type 1: Dry skin

Dry skin is very common, and it can be a major cause of skin problems like wrinkles, dryness and redness. Because of this, many people are looking for ways to combat dry skin. While genetics play an important role in how much moisture your skin holds, there are also other factors that can affect the natural moisture balance of your skin.

To understand how genetics affect dry skin, it's important to know where your natural oils come from in your body. You have two types of oil glands: sebaceous glands and apocrine glands. The sebaceous glands produce an oily substance called sebum that lubricates and protects the skin cells from rubbing against one another when they move around on the surface of your body; this helps keep them hydrated and keeps them from drying out. Apocrine glands produce a more viscous substance that helps keep hair follicles open so sweat can escape through them during perspiration (sweat).

Your genes also determine whether or not you produce enough sebum or apocrine sweat, as well as which type of oil gland you have (sebaceous or apocrine).

Skin Type 2: Oily skin

Having oily skin can be quite a struggle. The excess oil produced by your skin can lead to clogged pores and breakouts, making it challenging to maintain a clear complexion. However, did you know that your genetics play a significant role in determining your skin's oil production?

Your genetic makeup is unique to you, and it influences how your skin behaves. Several genes are involved in regulating sebum production, which contributes to oily skin. For example, the ELOVL gene is associated with increased sebum production, while the AQP5 gene [5] affects the water content in your skin and can impact oiliness.

Although scientists haven't pinpointed the exact causes of oily skin, they have identified several likely factors. Hormones also play a crucial role, with genes like AR, SRD5A2 and CYP17A1 influencing hormone levels that can affect sebum production. Additionally, factors like diet, stress, and lifestyle choices can further influence your skin's oiliness.

Understanding the genetic component of oily skin can provide valuable insights into managing and controlling excess oil production. By knowing your genetic predisposition, you can tailor your skincare routine and lifestyle choices accordingly. This may include using oil-control products, following a balanced diet, managing stress levels and adopting suitable skincare practices.

Skin type 3: Combination skin

The genes that determine whether you have combination or oily skin can be passed down from your parents, but the amount of oiliness you have will also be determined by your genes.

The genes that affect combination skin are mainly located on chromosome 17. The gene known as KITLG1 is responsible for making a protein called keratinocyte growth factor-like protein 1 (KGF1), which helps cells repair the damage and grow.

When people with combination skin have this gene, they usually have less sebum than those with oily skin. In addition, they tend to produce less of it and have less of a tendency to clog pores. This means that their skin is less prone to breakouts and blemishes, and it looks healthier overall.

Another gene family that is associated with combination skin is the HLA-DQB1*02, HLA-DQB1*03 and HLA-DQB1*06 genes. Combined, they make up a complex of genes that determine how your body produces melanin.

The combination of these three genes determines whether you have dry or oily skin. If you have dry skin and one of these three genes is defective, your skin will be dry and prone to flaking and cracking. If you have oily skin and one of these three genes is defective, then your skin will be oily with large pores, acne and blackheads.

If none of these three genes are working correctly, there will be no change in how much or how little oil your body produces.

YOU KNOW THE FAMOUS SAYING, 'YOU ARE WHAT YOU EAT'. WELL, IT'S TRUE.

Your genes can make or break your skin. Not a great thing if you want to look younger, but there's good news! You can have wonderful skin—deservedly, if not totally healthy—if you take control of your genes, nourish them, and keep them happy with lots of antioxidants and nutrients. Get ready for the best skincare diet tips and recipes!

Even though you're not a scientist and don't have access to your own DNA, you can still get the best advice on how genetics affect your skin.

THE SECRET?

The key lies in understanding the genetic traits passed down from your parents and how they impact your skin, a process that can be enhanced through genetic testing.

What makes beautiful skin? Genetics, most likely, but there's so much more to it! Just like how I'm blond and blue-eyed, your skin is genetically predisposed to be beautiful. But don't just let yourself accept these facts; instead, apply the right skincare tips and techniques to help your skin glow like a freaking space station.

There is no doubt that genetics play a major role in how healthy your skin looks, but it is also true that many factors can influence how well your skin responds to those genes. There are some things you can do to increase the health of your skin.

WRAP YOUR MIND AROUND THE IMPORTANCE OF GOOD GENES

It can be frustrating to find one surefire way to make your skin glow. That's because the genes that give you healthy, youthful-looking skin are a little bit like the genes for blue eyes: they're all over the place.

In fact, there are two different types of genes that affect how your skin looks and feels, according to a recent study published in *Scientific Reports*. The findings suggest that there may be more than one gene responsible for glowing skin.

The first is called HIF1a. It's responsible for making proteins called hyaluronan (HA), which are basically water-binding proteins that help keep your skin plump and hydrated. HA is what gives your skin its bouncy look and feel.

The second is SIRT1, which helps regulate cell metabolism in order to maintain the health and function of cells throughout life. SIRT1 also controls the expression of other genes involved in ageing and protecting from oxidative stress—basically, it keeps yours looking good as time goes on!

Genetics can make a big difference in how you look, but they are just one factor in the way you look and your overall health.

CHAPTER 8

HYDRATION 101

Skincare is one of the most important things you can do to make your skin healthy and radiant.

You may think that the best way to look younger is by getting Botox or other extreme procedures, but this is not always true.

Imagine your skin as a desert, longing for a refreshing oasis. Hydration acts as that magical oasis, quenching the thirst of your skin cells. It helps maintain elasticity, preventing the appearance of fine lines and wrinkles. Say goodbye to parched skin and hello to a youthful, plump complexion!

We've all experienced those dull days when our skin seems to have lost its spark. Fear not! Hydration comes to the rescue, banishing dullness and bringing forth a vibrant, revitalized complexion.

So, why is hydration so important for your skin? Well, let me break it down for you:

First off, keeping your skin hydrated is like giving it a big drink of water. When your skin is well hydrated, it stays plump and bouncy. It helps maintain a nice balance of moisture, so your skin looks smooth and supple. Who doesn't want that?

Not only that, but hydration also helps with the elasticity of your skin. Think of it like a rubber band. When your skin is hydrated, it's all stretchy and flexible. That means fewer wrinkles and sagging. So, keeping your skin hydrated can help you look younger and fresher.

But it's not just about looks. Hydration also plays a role in nourishing your skin. When your skin is hydrated, it gets all the good stuff it needs, like nutrients and oxygen. It helps your skin cells regenerate and repair themselves, which is super important for keeping your skin healthy and vibrant.

Speaking of looks, hydrated skin has a better tone and texture. Dehydrated skin can look dull and rough, which is no fun. But when you keep your skin hydrated, it looks brighter and smoother. Plus, it helps maintain a nice balance of oils, so you don't end up with a greasy or dry mess on your face.

Hydration actually strengthens your skin's protective barrier. It's like armour against all the bad stuff in the environment. When your skin is dehydrated, this armour gets weak, and your skin becomes more sensitive and prone to irritation. But if you keep your skin hydrated, it stays strong and can fight off those irritants.

HOW TO KEEP YOUR SKIN HYDRATED

The **second step** to healthy skin is to **drink a lot of water**. Aim for around eight glasses a day. Water is the most important nutrient for your body and helps flush toxins out of your cells, keeping them healthy.

Eat foods rich in antioxidants. Antioxidants protect cells from free radicals that cause damage to skin cells, which can lead to wrinkles and age spots. Foods high in antioxidants include dark leafy greens, berries, citrus fruits and red wine—but don't overdo it! Too many antioxidants can actually be harmful to your skin by causing dryness or irritation in sensitive areas like the eyes or lips.

Want to power up your regular water intake?

Want to combine the benefits of a 2-in-1 drink?

Have a glass of ANTIOXIDANT WATER

Fruit and vegetable water is one of the best things you can do for your skin. These types of waters are packed with vitamins and minerals that are essential for healthy skin cells. They also contain antioxidants, which help prevent free radicals from harming your skin cells.

Add some cut fruits or vegetables from the list below to level up your hydration status:

- Strawberries and kiwi
- Fresh ginger
- Pineapple
- Watermelon and mint leaves
- Apple and cinnamon
- Orange and cucumber
- Cucumber, lemon and mint leaves

Another way to keep your skin hydrated is by **drinking cold tea or herbal detox tea by Nutracy Lifestyle** after meals. This helps cool down your body temperature and will help you cool off when you get hot during exercise or after being outside in the sun all day long!

However, drinking too much water can also cause bloating and headaches. If you're still thirsty after drinking quarts of water a day, consider cutting back a little bit or switching your beverage of choice.

It is easy for people to forget about their hydration needs, especially when they're busy with work or school. But drinking more water could help you look younger and more vibrant than ever before. In fact, the best way to fight dry, dull skin is with hydration and nourishment!

Myth: Drinking caffeinated beverages like coffee and tea dehydrates the skin.

Fact: While caffeine is a mild diuretic, meaning it may increase urine production, moderate consumption of caffeinated beverages doesn't lead to significant dehydration or negatively impact skin hydration. The water content in these beverages still contributes to your overall fluid intake. However, excessive consumption of caffeinated drinks may have a diuretic effect, so it's best to balance your fluid intake with plain water or hydrating beverages.

CHAPTER 9

ESSENTIAL NUTRIENTS FOR GLOWING SKIN

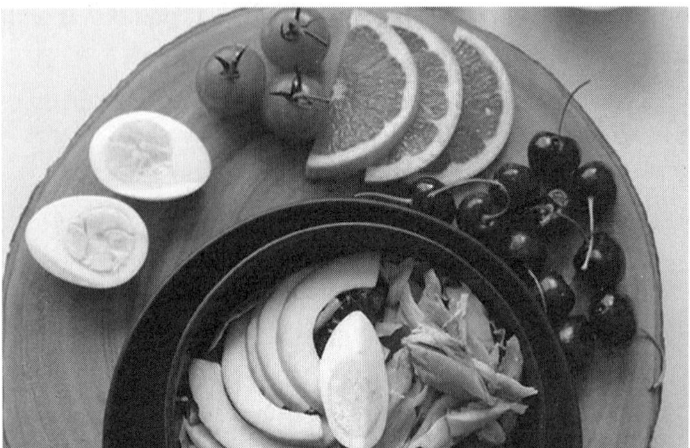

Good nutrition is important to keep the body's metabolism functioning smoothly and organs healthy. What you consume has a big impact on your skin's health and ageing. As a result, nutrients that promote healthy, beautiful skin must be included in your daily diet. To appear, work, and feel well, your skin requires the appropriate combination of nutrients. Essential nutrition is essential for maintaining healthy skin. The food you eat provides the building blocks and nutrients necessary for the growth, repair, and function of your skin cells.

You can unlock the secret to radiant skin through the power of good nutrition! Discover the perfect combination of nutrients that will unleash the beauty within and nourish your skin from the inside out. By embracing a daily diet rich in skin-enhancing elements, you'll witness the transformation of your complexion, as it becomes a glowing testament to the benefits of proper nourishment. Prepare to embark on a journey where every bite you take brings you closer to the vibrant, youthful skin you've always dreamed of.

Here are some key reasons why good nutrition is important for skin health:

- **Nutrient supply:** A well-balanced diet that includes a variety of fruits, vegetables, whole grains, lean proteins, good quality protein, and healthy fats ensures that your skin receives essential vitamins, minerals and antioxidants. These nutrients play a crucial role in promoting skin health and addressing common skin concerns.
- **Skin hydration:** Proper hydration is important for maintaining skin health. Drinking an adequate amount of water helps keep your skin hydrated, plump and supple. It also supports the function of the skin's natural barrier, which helps prevent moisture loss and protects against external irritants.

- **Collagen production:** Collagen is a protein that provides structure and elasticity to the skin. Consuming foods rich in collagen-boosting nutrients, such as vitamin C, vitamin A, copper and proline, can help support collagen synthesis and maintain skin firmness and elasticity.
- **Protection against oxidative stress:** The skin is constantly exposed to environmental stressors, such as pollution and UV radiation, which can generate free radicals. Free radicals are unstable molecules that can cause cellular damage and accelerate skin ageing. Antioxidant-rich foods, such as berries, leafy greens, citrus fruits, and nuts, help neutralize free radicals and protect the skin from oxidative stress.
- **Reduction of inflammation:** Inflammation is a common factor in many skin conditions, including acne, eczema, and psoriasis. Certain nutrients, such as omega-3 fatty acids, vitamin E, and zinc, have anti-inflammatory properties and can help reduce skin inflammation. Consuming a diet rich in these nutrients may support healthier skin and alleviate inflammatory skin conditions.
- **Wound healing:** Proper nutrition is vital for the healing of wounds and the prevention of scars. Nutrients like vitamin C, vitamin E, zinc, and protein are important for collagen synthesis, tissue repair, and immune function, all of which contribute to effective wound healing.
- **Overall skin appearance:** Your diet can impact the overall appearance of your skin. Nutrient deficiencies or a diet

high in processed foods and sugar can contribute to skin problems like acne, dullness, and premature ageing. On the other hand, a nutrient-dense diet that includes plenty of fruits, vegetables, whole grains, and lean proteins can help promote clear, radiant, and youthful-looking skin.

While good nutrition is important for skin health, it's important to note that individual skin types and conditions may have specific dietary considerations.

Let's understand the building blocks of skin; the main responsible nutrients essential for the glowing and nourishing skin barrier!

(1) Protein

Proteins play a crucial role in maintaining skin health through various mechanisms. These include:

- **Collagen production:** Collagen is the most abundant protein in the skin and plays a vital role in maintaining its structure, elasticity and strength. Proteins provide the necessary amino acids for collagen synthesis, which helps in wound healing, skin regeneration, and maintaining a youthful appearance.
- **Tissue repair and regeneration:** Proteins are essential for the repair and regeneration of skin tissues. When the skin is damaged due to injuries, cuts, or burns, proteins help in the formation of new skin cells and the production of collagen to heal the damaged area.

- **Moisture retention:** Proteins contribute to maintaining the skin's natural moisture balance. They help create a protective barrier on the skin's surface, preventing excessive water loss and keeping the skin hydrated. This helps to improve skin texture, reduce dryness, and minimize the appearance of fine lines and wrinkles.
- **Antioxidant defense:** Some proteins in the skin act as antioxidants, protecting it from damage caused by free radicals. Free radicals are unstable molecules that can cause oxidative stress and accelerate skin ageing. Proteins with antioxidant properties neutralize these free radicals, reducing oxidative damage and promoting healthier-looking skin.
- **Immune function:** Proteins play a role in the immune response of the skin. They help in the production of antibodies, which fight against pathogens and protect the skin from infections. A healthy immune system contributes to overall skin health and faster healing of skin issues.

Your body converts the proteins you eat into amino acids, which then recycles to generate other proteins like collagen and keratin, which make up the structure of your skin. Some amino acids are antioxidants that protect skin cells from UV radiation and free radicals produced by the body when certain meals are broken down.

Imagine the proteins you eat as superheroes arriving at a bustling construction site. They get to work, transforming into powerful amino acids that become the foundation for building structures like collagen and keratin in your skin. These superhero proteins ensure your skin is strong and sturdy, like a protective shield.

But wait, there's more! Some of these amino acid superheroes have an extra superpower—they're antioxidants. They swoop in just in time to protect your skin cells from the evil villains known as free radicals and harmful UV radiation. These villains can cause damage and lead to skin problems. Thankfully, the antioxidant amino acids save the day, keeping your skin safe and radiant.

So, by including protein-packed foods in your diet, you provide your body with the heroes it needs to construct and defend your skin's health. It's like having a team of superheroes working tirelessly to keep your skin strong, resilient, and ready to take on the world.

Below are the sources of proteins for its absorption:

Vegetarian Sources of Protein	Non-Vegetarian Sources of Protein
• Greek yoghurt • Lentils • Cottage cheese • Hemp seeds • Chia seeds • Edamame • Green peas • Quinoa	• Egg whites • Chicken breast • Chicken liver • Salmon • Sardines • Tuna • Prawns • Shrimps

• Peanut butter • Almonds • Firm tofu • Low fat yoghurt • Squash and pumpkin seeds • Mushrooms, peas, beans,legumes • Seitan • Kidney beans • Chickpeas	

(2) Vitamin A

Vitamin A protects against UV damage by decreasing the breakdown of collagen. It also keeps your skin from becoming dry and itchy. This anti-ageing vitamin aids in the prevention of clogged pores, enhances skin tone, and stimulates collagen formation. This fat-soluble vitamin is often found in foods and supplements in the form of beta-carotene. It is a powerful antioxidant that is widely found in sunscreens, anti-ageing serums, moisturizers and other cosmetics. Vitamin A not only promotes moisturized, young skin, but it can also aid in the treatment of acne.

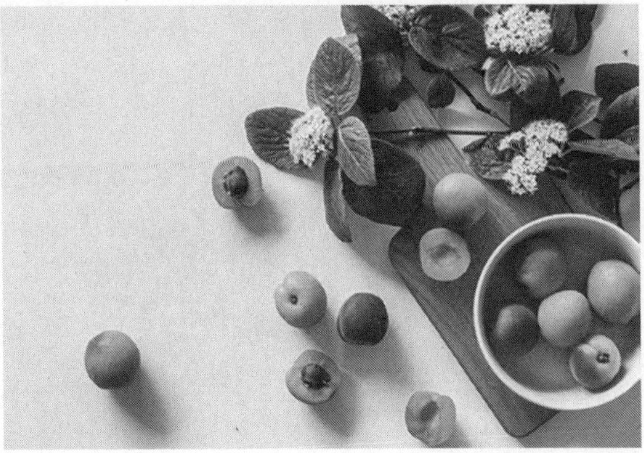

(3) B Vitamins

Benefits	Sources
• Promotes cell development and renewal, which rejuvenates both the upper and bottom layers of your skin (dermis and epidermis) • Collagen synthesis is increased, which smoothes the skin and reduces fine lines and wrinkles. • Scavenges free radicals on your skin, reducing damage caused by the sun's damaging UV rays • Promotes faster wound healing and strengthens the skin's inherent immune system	• Orange or yellow vegetables and fruits such as carrots, pumpkins, yellow bell pepper, oranges, papaya, mangoes, etc. • Green leafy vegetables such as spinach, broccoli, etc. • Cod liver oil, eggs, beef liver, etc. • Fortified milk and other dairy products like cheese, ice cream, etc.

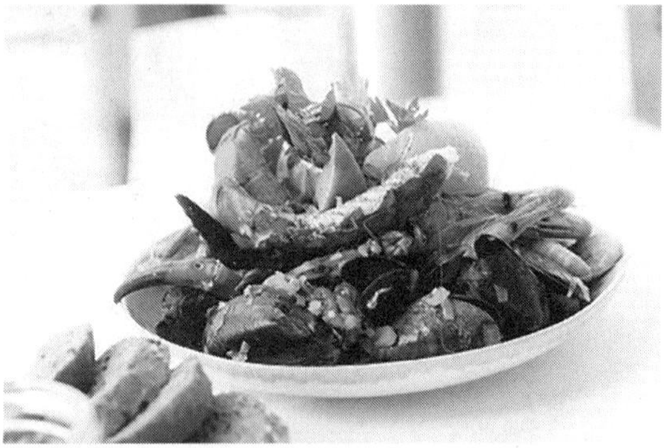

B Vitamins	Benefits	Sources
Vitamin B	Vitamin B is also an excellent skin-lightening agent. Your hyperpigmentation will fade with time if you use it on a daily basis.	Meat (especially liver), seafood, poultry, eggs, dairy products, legumes, leafy greens, seeds, and fortified foods, such as breakfast cereal and nutritional yeast
Vitamin B2	These vitamins are helpful for dry skin or acne since they can help enhance skin tone, make skin more vibrant, and regulate natural oils.	Milk, yoghurt, cheese, eggs, lean beef and pork, organ meats (beef liver), chicken breast, salmon, etc.

B Vitamins	Benefits	Sources
Vitamin B3	Vitamin B3 enhances the surface structure of aged skin by smoothing out the skin's texture and reducing wrinkles.	Red meat (beef, beef liver, pork), poultry, fish, brown rice, fortified cereals and breads, nuts, seeds, legumes, bananas, etc.
Vitamin B6	This B vitamin aids in the reduction of the negative consequences of hormonal imbalance, which can result in acne breakouts. Take on hormonal acne, inflammation, and redness with B6.	Pork, poultry, such as chicken or turkey, peanuts, soya beans, wheat germ, oats, bananas, etc.
Vitamin B12	Vitamin B12 deficiency causes skin to become dull and tired (it reduces dark spots and discolouration which can make skin tone uneven).	Meat, fish, milk, cheese, eggs, fortified breakfast cereals, etc.

B Vitamins	Benefits	Sources
	It plays a crucial role in reducing dark spots and uneven skin tone, giving your skin a more vibrant and balanced look. By ensuring an adequate intake of vitamin B12, you can help maintain a healthy, glowing complexion and promote skin that feels nourished and refreshed.	

(4) Vitamin C

Vitamin C protects the skin against free radicals and reduces the risk of skin cancer. Vitamin C deficiency can lead to easy bruising, bleeding gums, and slow-healing ulcers. Vitamin C products are high in antioxidants, which are known to give our skin a brightening and glowy appearance. It fights symptoms of ageing and UV exposure, as well as hyperpigmentation and dark areas, to improve the appearance of skin naturally. This water-soluble vitamin, also known as ascorbic acid, is found in significant concentrations in the skin of healthy people.

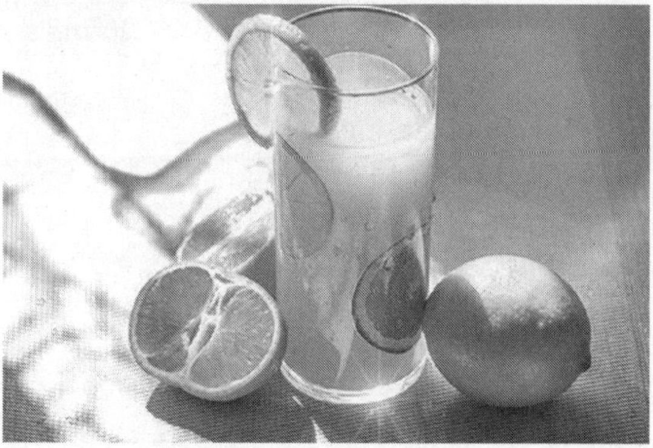

Benefits	Sources
• Vitamin C helps to protect your skin in a variety of ways. Although vitamin C deficiency is uncommon, it can have serious consequences for your skin. • Vitamin C is essential for the healthy functioning of the immune system and aids in the reduction of inflammation. • It's also a potent antioxidant that could help prevent skin cancer. • It encourages collagen formation, which keeps your skin tight and aids in the healing of wounds and scars.	Citrus fruits such as lemons, tangerine, grapefruit, etc. Tomatoes, green andred peppers, green vegetables like broccoli, etc. Other fruits such as kiwi, strawberries, cantaloupes, etc.

Benefits	Sources
• Vitamin C supplementation may also aid in preventing photodamage produced by the sun's damaging UV radiation. Vitamin C is necessary for a healthy complexion and even skin tone.	

(5) Vitamin D

When your skin is exposed to direct sunshine for a few minutes each day, your body can create vitamin D. Vitamin D is a vital nutrient that plays a crucial role in supporting the health of your skin. When your skin is exposed to sunlight, it has the incredible ability to produce vitamin D, which is essential for various skin functions. This nutrient helps regulate the growth and differentiation of skin cells, ensuring the proper formation and maturation of the outermost layer of your skin. By promoting healthy cell turnover, vitamin D contributes to a smooth and balanced complexion. Additionally, vitamin D possesses anti-inflammatory properties that can soothe skin inflammation and promote a calm and radiant appearance. It's important to maintain sufficient levels of vitamin D through sunlight exposure, consumption of vitamin-D-rich foods like fatty fish and fortified products or supplementation if necessary, in order to support optimal skin health.

Benefits	Sources
• Enhances the skin's barrier function, protecting it from bacteria and hazardous substances • Prevents dryness of the skin by locking in moisture. • Boosts the formation of immune system cells in the skin, which improves skin immunity • Controls immune cell activity to prevent the immune system from becoming overactive • Has anti-bacterial properties when applied to the skin • Regulates oil production through the skin's sebaceous glands	• Dairy products such as milk, butter, cheese, etc. • Eggs, fish, fish liver oil • Fortified plant-based milk, yoghurt, juices and breakfast cereals to which recommended amount of vitamin D has been added

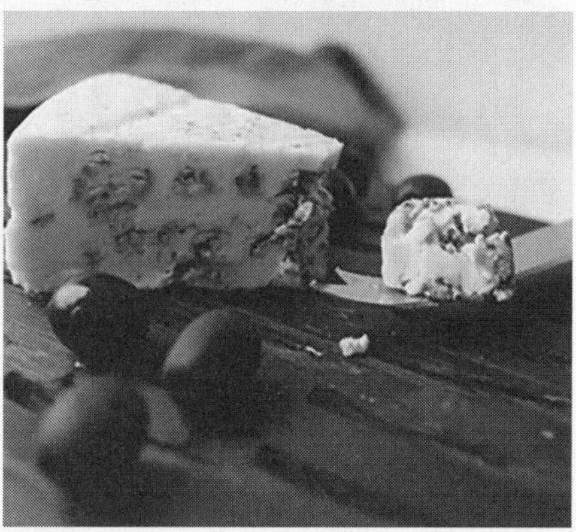

(6) Vitamin E

Vitamin E is an antioxidant and anti-inflammatory substance that may absorb UV light's energy, which causes skin damage such as wrinkles, drooping and skin cancer. It aids in the function of vitamin C, which is to reinforce cell membranes. Vitamin E is commonly used to cure scarring, and it can also be used to brighten dark areas. It hydrates and nourishes the skin. It improves your skin's radiance and makes it smooth and healthy. In addition to preserving skin health, the oil is believed to minimize hyperpigmentation and wrinkles. This fat-soluble vitamin has anti-inflammatory and antioxidant effects. When administered topically, it is known as the 'magic potion' for healthy, bright skin. However, the best source of this skin-friendly nutrient is a diet high in vitamin E.

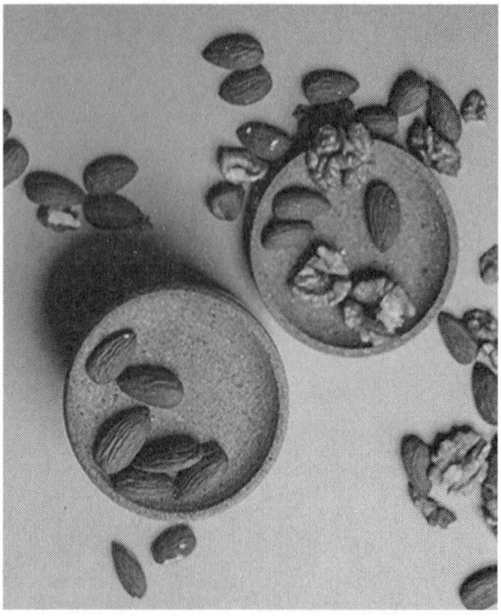

Benefits	Sources
• Keeps skin moisturized, thus preventing dryness and irritation • Protects skin from damage due to the UV rays of the sun • Helps to reduce dark spots and wrinkles • Makes your skin look smooth and refreshed	• Nuts such as almonds (very high content), hazelnuts, peanuts, etc. • Vegetable oils from wheat germ, sunflower, safflower, etc. • Fortified foods such as breakfast cereals, spreads, etc.

(7) Biotin

Biotin gives dull and aged skin a naturally renewed appearance, making it a good choice for them. This vitamin aids in maintaining the mucous membranes of the skin. Biotin also plays a crucial role in the process of metabolizing fat, which is essential for maintaining healthy skin.

Benefits	Sources
• Biotin produces fatty acids that nourish the skin to maintain a clear complexion. When the protective outer layer of skin is unbalanced, dry and dehydrated skin can manifest.	• Egg yolk, organ meats (liver, kidney), nuts like almonds, peanuts, pecans and walnuts • Nut butters, soybeans and other legumes • Whole grains and cereals • Cauliflower, bananas and mushrooms

• It assists in the production of new cells and helps oil glands function properly, resulting in the healthy condition of skin.	

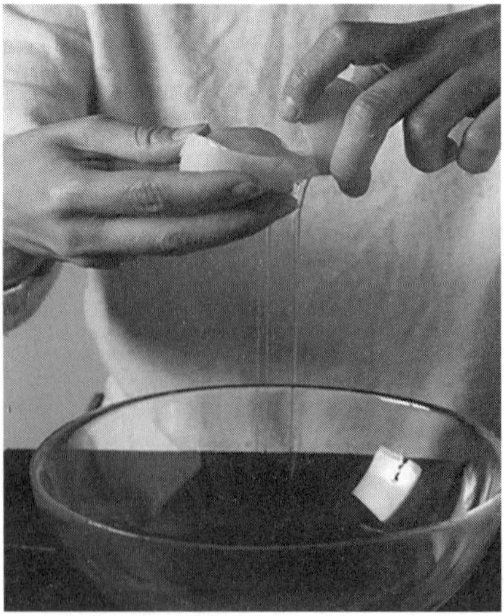

(8) Calcium

Another micronutrient, specifically a mineral, found in dairy products that helps to maintain a healthy skin glow is calcium. This vitamin is stored in the epidermis, the skin's outermost layer, and controls sebum production to keep the skin moisturized and free of eczema.

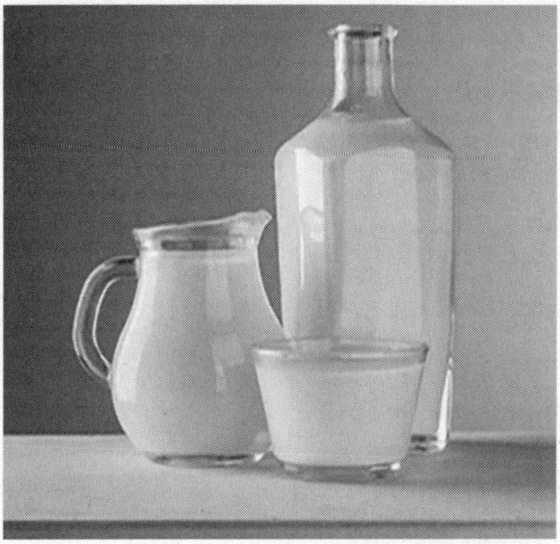

Benefits	Sources
• **Natural moisturizer**: Calcium occupies a large mass of our body materials. Skin becomes dry, wrinkled and itchy without its required intake. Calcium works with the epidermis to produce sebum, a natural skin-coating substance that keeps the skin to maintain its natural moisture. Inadequate amount of calcium produces less sebum leaving the skin dry and unhealthy. People may face serious skin disorders like eczema in case of dry and damaged skin and this can even lead to skin cancer.	• Milk • Cheese and other dairy foods • Green leafy vegetables, such as curly kale, okra, but not spinach (spinach does contain high levels of calcium, but the body cannot digest it all) • Soya drinks with added calcium • Bread • Anything made with fortified flour

Benefits	Sources
• **Skin pH Balance:** Calcium is essential for regulating the skin's pH balance. Maintaining the appropriate pH level is crucial for a healthy skin barrier function, which helps protect against environmental stressors, bacteria, and other harmful substances. A balanced pH level also supports the skin's natural defense mechanisms, promoting overall skin health and resilience. • **Skin renewal:** Calcium is responsible for proper cell turnover, but it would not be possible without the correct calcium dosage. It ensures the renewal of skin and removes dead cells by creating protective lipid barriers. • **Antioxidant:** Though calcium itself is not an antioxidant, it plays a major role in the production of antioxidants that prevent DNA damage and amazingly protect our skin texture.	

Benefits	Sources
• **Protection against harsh weather conditions:** Cold or frosting weather always affects the skin. Its proper and required intake protects your skin from harsh weather conditions. Dry and itchy skin can be successfully warded off with the magic of calcium, as it offers protective epidermal tissues against dry or harsh weather. • **Reduces stress:** It soothes the nervous system and reduces stress and depression. An adequate amount of this mineral considerably reduces the risk of damage to elastin and collagen.	

(9) Copper

Copper has two important features that make it a good active component for products that come into contact with the skin and are intended to promote the skin's health. Copper is important for skin protein production and stability, as well as having biocidal effects.

Benefits of Copper	Sources
• **Reduced appearance of wrinkles:** Studies of copper peptides have shown that they can help reduce the appearance of fine lines and wrinkles by increasing collagen proteins. Over time, collagen may help to 'plump up' your skin, reducing the appearance of wrinkles.	Oysters and other shellfish
• **Firmer skin**: In addition to increased collagen production, copper peptides are also said to help boost elastin proteins. This may help create firmer and smoother skin.	Whole grains, beans, nuts, potatoes, and organ meats (kidneys and liver)
• **Even skin tone**: Copper peptides stand out from other types of peptides because of their ability to potentially repair your skin and even out your skin tone. It's thought that copper peptides may potentially remove damaged connective tissues from your skin while adding new ones at the same time. This may reduce the appearance of sunspots (also called age spots), acne, scars and other causes of uneven skin tone.	Dark leafy greens, dried fruits, such as prunes and cocoa, black pepper, and yeast
• **Antioxidant effects:** Copper peptides may also have antioxidant effects on the skin, which may reduce inflammation and prevent further damage.	

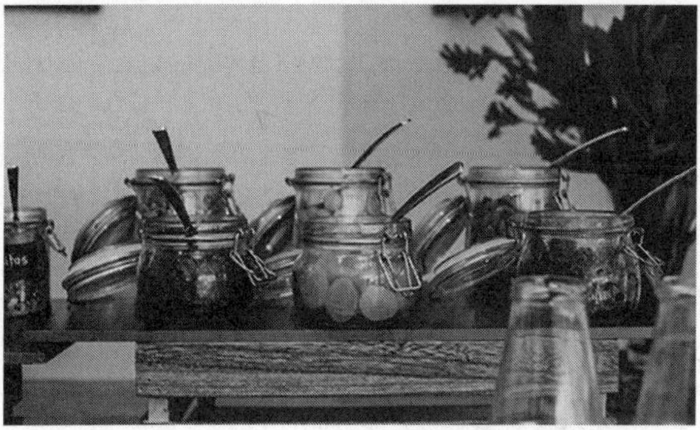

(10) Cysteine

L-cysteine is an antioxidant with anti-ageing properties for the skin. Following the discovery of its anti-melanogenic capabilities, the glutathione component has become a potential skin-lightening factor. L-cysteine, an antioxidant and amino acid, offers anti-ageing benefits for the skin. It contains glutathione, which has potential skin-lightening properties by inhibiting melanin production. L-cysteine's antioxidant properties help combat free radicals, preventing premature ageing and skin damage. Additionally, it supports collagen synthesis, promoting skin firmness and reducing the appearance of wrinkles. Although not directly used in skincare products, including L-cysteine-rich foods in your diet can support glutathione production and contribute to overall skin health.

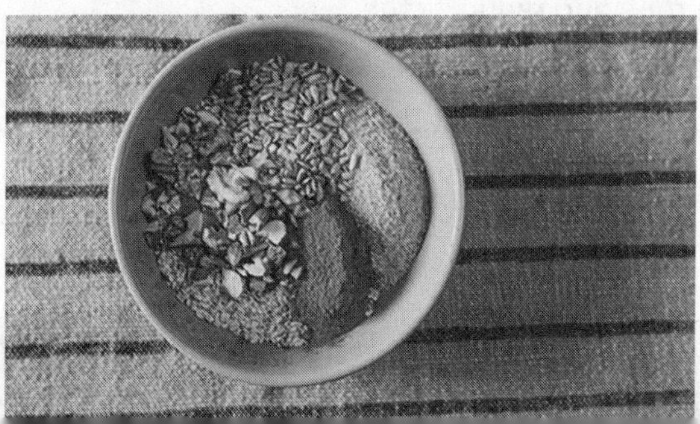

Benefits	Sources
• Cysteine helps reduce the effects of ageing on the skin. • The skewing of the melanin synthesis pathway towards the generation of lighter pheomelanin instead of darker eumelanin, resulting in a lightening effect, has been proposed as one mechanism of action to explain this feature. • One way that L-cysteine may help lighten the skin is by shifting the production of melanin, the pigment responsible for skin colour, towards a lighter form called pheomelanin instead of the darker form called eumelanin. • This change in melanin synthesis can contribute to a lightening effect on the skin. This is one of the ways that L-cysteine is thought to work in promoting a more even skin tone and reducing the appearance of dark spots or hyperpigmentation.	Chicken, turkey, yoghurt, cheese, eggs, sunflower seeds and legumes

(11) Iron

Haemoglobin levels drop as a result of a lack of iron, which leads to a reduction in red blood cells (RBCs). Reduced oxygen flow might cause your skin to lose its colour and seem sallow. Your skin can shine with a healthy intake of iron-rich foods in your regular diet.

Iron is like the superhero that keeps our skin healthy and glowing. It does some amazing things for our skin! Firstly, it helps carry oxygen to our skin cells, making sure they stay happy and full of life. Secondly, it helps in repairing and growing new skin cells, so our skin can stay fresh and vibrant. Iron also plays a big role in making collagen, which is like the scaffolding that keeps our skin firm and bouncy. When we get a cut or a scrape, iron jumps in to help with healing by creating new blood vessels and collagen at the injured spot.

Did you know iron even helps with our skin's colour? It's involved in making melanin, which protects us from the sun's rays and gives our skin an even tone. So, let's make sure we get enough iron through a healthy diet to keep our skin looking and feeling its best!

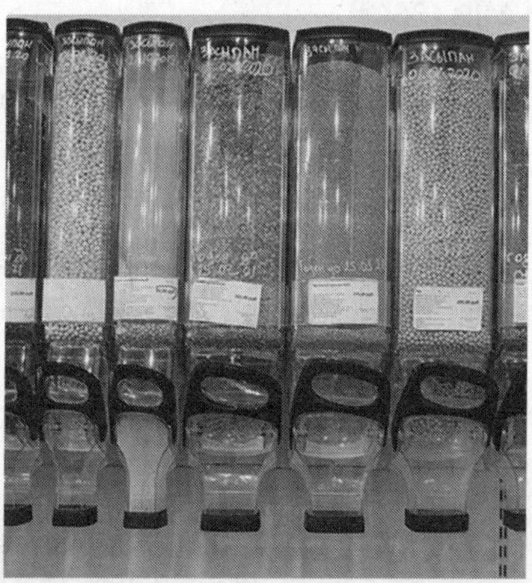

Benefits	Sources
• **Reduces dark spots and under-eye circles:** These are usually caused by anaemic conditions wherein less than the required amount of oxygenated blood reaches the blood vessels on the surface of the skin and under the eyes. With iron consumption, the body is able to send enough oxygenated blood to these parts. This helps to reduce dark spots and under-eye dark circles. • **Improving the glow of skin:** The bright pinkish glow that some people have on their skin is due to a healthy amount of red blood cells (RBCs) and is one of the many benefits of iron in the body.	• Liver, red meat, beans, such as red kidney beans, edamame beans and chickpeas • Nuts, dried fruit, such as dried apricots, fortified breakfast cereals and soybean flour

(12) Methionine

Methionine (L-methionine) is an important amino acid found in food as well as a dietary supplement. It is an essential amino acid that improves skin brightness and glow. It is required for regular human tissue growth and repair and cannot be produced by the body; hence, it is considered an essential amino acid.

Benefits	Sources
• The sulphur in methionine nourishes skin. • Protects the skin cells from pollutants • Facilitates the detoxifying process, thus helping to glow • Slows down the ageing process	• Eggs, meat and fish • Sesame seeds, Brazil nuts, and some other plant seeds, and cereal grains

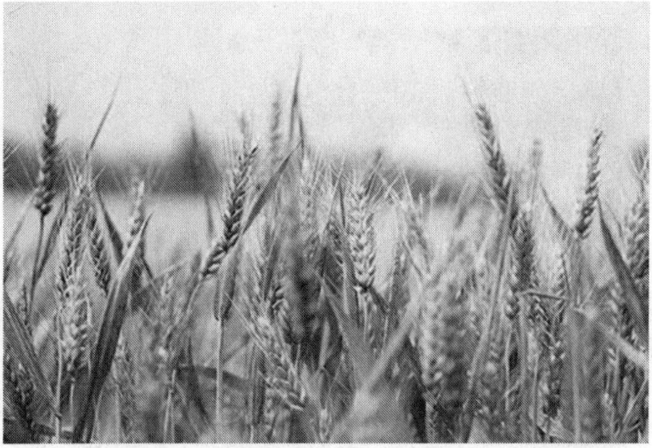

(13) Potassium

Potassium promotes cell renewal at a higher rate. Another advantage of potassium for skin is that it promotes quick cell proliferation. This feature makes your skin look younger, healthier, and more radiant. Additionally, newer cell growth is quite beneficial for removing scars and imperfections from the skin's surface.

Potassium plays a vital role in promoting faster cell renewal and proliferation, which contributes to youthful and radiant skin. Its ability to accelerate cell growth helps rejuvenate the skin, making it appear healthier and more vibrant. Furthermore, the increased cell turnover facilitated by potassium can aid in reducing the visibility of scars and imperfections on the skin's surface. By incorporating potassium-rich foods into your diet, you can harness the benefits of this mineral for maintaining a rejuvenated and flawless complexion.

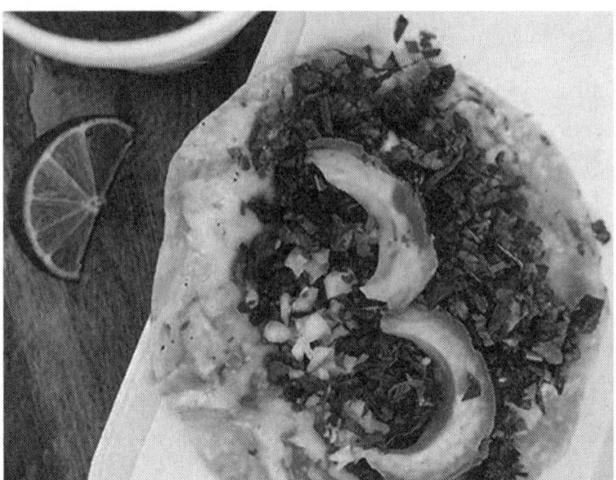

Benefits	Sources
• **Prevents dry skin:** If your skin constantly feels dry and parched despite applying topical moisturizers and skincare products, then there is a chance that you might be deficient in potassium. Potassium helps regulate the water storage in your body and prevents moisture loss, which in turn keeps your skin healthy and glowing. • **Promotes faster cell renewal:** Another benefit of potassium for skin is that it supports the rapid growth of new cells. This function helps your skin look young, healthy and glowing. Additionally, newer cell growth is really useful to quickly eliminate scars and blemishes from the surface of your skin.	• Dried fruits (raisins and apricots) • Beans, lentils, potatoes and winter squash (acorn and butternut) • Spinach, broccoli, beet greens, avocado and bananas

Benefits	Sources
• **Helps maintain skin's pH balance:** If you have really dry skin, your skin's pH balance could be disrupted. This could lead to several skin problems, dryness and a compromised skin barrier being the most prevalent. But since potassium is an excellent way to prevent dry skin, it works really well in maintaining your skin's pH balance and keeping it healthy for a longer period of time.	

(14) Selenium

Selenium is another mineral that keeps skin firm and protected. Selenium protects the skin from free radical damage, preventing wrinkles from forming prematurely. It also aids in the prevention of UV damage, inflammation, and pigmentation in cell membranes.

Benefits	Sources
• **Prevents signs of ageing:** Selenium fights free radicals, minimizes skin damage and inflammation, and may even prevent skin cancer.	Seafood, organ meats, Brazil nuts, breads, cereals, poultry, red meat and eggs

Benefits	Sources
• **Reduces inflammation:** Inflammation is caused by ultraviolet rays, stress, a poor diet and lack of minerals. Selenium fights inflammatory cytokines that eventually cause skin damage. • **Benefits the immune system:** White blood cells are micro-soldiers on the front lines of immune defence. Selenium boosts white blood cell function, preventing both bacterial skin infections and viruses. • **Promotes skin healing and reduces acne:** Selenium (when paired with vitamin E) boosts glutathione, which may help skin heal. What's more, selenium can decrease the incidence of acne.	

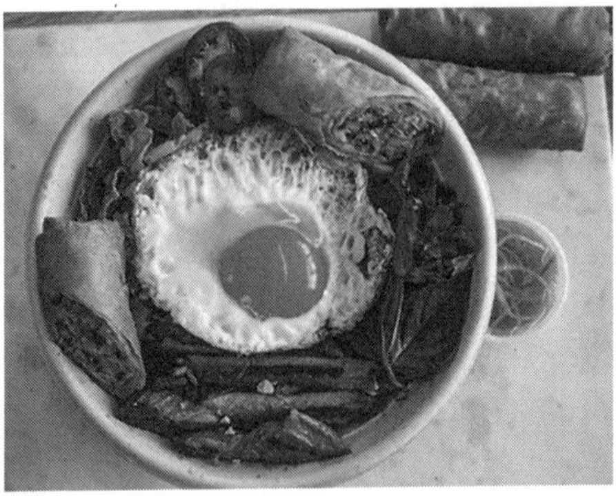

(15) Silica

Silica gives a glow since it is a strong oxygen transporter and improves the flow of both nutrients and oxygen to the skin. It allows red blood cells to carry 20 per cent more oxygen, which keeps the skin moisturized.

Benefits	Sources
• Silica also promotes the production of collagen, which is your body's most abundant protein. Collagen is responsible for helping your skin maintain its youthfulness by keeping it firm and elastic. It also reduces the appearance of fine lines and wrinkles.	Green beans, leafy greens, brown rice, cereals and lentils

Benefits	Sources
• Silica helps sun-damaged skin, as with 10 mg of silica on a daily basis, the skin's rough texture gets improved. • Silica has anti-inflammatory properties as it helps to relieve symptoms like acne. Additionally, it is also great for sensitive skin as it carries a lot of oxygen, which gives the skin radiance.	

(16) Zinc

Zinc contains antioxidants, which help fight the free radicals present in our body and also effectively delay skin ageing. Antioxidants help make the skin youthful and glowy. Regular yet limited consumption of this essential mineral can also help in preventing acne, dullness and dryness in the skin.

Benefits	Sources
• Zinc aids in the healing of wounds on the skin. Because of how it interacts with other nutrients in your body, such as iron, it protects your skin from UV damage.	Whole grains and milk products Oysters, red meat and poultry

Benefits	Sources
It also has antioxidant properties. Zinc includes antioxidants, which aid in the battle against free radicals in our bodies and successfully prevent the ageing of our skin. Antioxidants contribute to the skin's youthfulness and radiance. • This vital mineral can also aid in preventing acne, dullness, and dryness in the skin when consumed in moderation.	Baked beans, chickpeas and nuts (such as cashews and almonds)

(17) Lycopene

Lycopene is a naturally occurring pigment and powerful antioxidant that provides foods with their vibrant colour and offers potential health benefits. Lycopene is known for its ability to protect the skin from UV damage, reduce oxidative stress, support collagen production, and promote a healthy, radiant complexion.

(18) Resveratrol

Resveratrol, a naturally occurring compound found in certain plants, has gained significant attention for its potential benefits to human health, particularly in relation to skin. With its antioxidant, anti-ageing and anti-inflammatory properties, resveratrol holds promise as a valuable ingredient for skincare. Derived from sources like grapes and berries, resveratrol offers protection against environmental damage, promotes cellular repair, improves skin elasticity, and helps reduce inflammation. Whether consumed through dietary sources or applied topically in skincare products, resveratrol presents an intriguing avenue for supporting skin health and enhancing the youthful appearance of the skin.

Benefits
• **Antioxidant protection:** Resveratrol is a potent antioxidant that helps neutralize harmful free radicals, protecting skin cells from oxidative stress and damage. This antioxidant activity helps to combat premature ageing and maintain theoverall health and integrity of the skin
• **Anti-ageing effects:** Resveratrol activates proteins called sirtuins, which play a role in regulating cellular processes related to ageing. By stimulating sirtuins, resveratrol promotes cellular repair and rejuvenation, helping to reducethe appearance of fine lines, wrinkles, and other signs of ageing.
• **Anti-inflammatory properties:** Chronic inflammation in theskin can contribute to various skin issues, such as acne, eczema, and psoriasis. Resveratrol possesses anti-inflammatory properties that help calm and soothe the skin, reducing the redness, irritation and inflammation associated with these conditions.

- **Protection against UV damage:**

Resveratrol has been foundto provide photoprotective effects, helping to shield the skin from the damaging effects of

Sources

Resveratrol is a compound found in various plant sources, particularly in the skin of grapes, berries, and peanuts. Here's a list of common sources of resveratrol:

1. Grapes (especially red grapes)
2. Red wine
3. Blueberries
4. Cranberries
5. Strawberries
6. Raspberries
7. Mulberries
8. Peanuts
9. Dark chocolate

The best diet for your skin is the one that works for you. Your diet can help you achieve a beautiful, healthy glow by promoting healthy cells, reducing inflammation and boosting collagen production.

Chapter 10

CRUCIAL SKIN-GLOW FOODS

- **Walnuts**: Walnuts are a good source of the essential fatty acids omega-3 and omega-6, which help fight the potential inflammatory response to excessive omega-6. They also contain zinc, which is essential for your skin to function properly as a barrier to bacteria and inflammation.

- **Pomegranate:** Pomegranate is what you need, especially if you walk in the sun too much. Not just the fruit but also its peels are rich in antioxidants, vitamins C, K, folate, and minerals, which help reduce UV damage and pigmentation and aid skin rejuvenation.

- **Muskmelon:** Muskmelon is packed with vitamins A, C, and K, folate, and minerals that are essential for good skin health. It has antioxidants and anti-inflammatory properties that help reduce skin issues like pigmentation.

- **Soybean**: Soybean contains isoflavones that block oestrogen, thereby reducing the appearance of wrinkles and improving skin elasticity. Isoflavones prevent dry skin and increase collagen production to improve skin texture; they can benefit women the most in the post-menopausal phase. They also protect your skin from UV radiation, preventing certain kinds of skin cancer.

- **Beetroot:** Beetroot contains huge amounts of vitamins and minerals that enhance the skin's glow. It has anti-inflammatory properties that prevent the outburst of acne and pimples. Including beetroot in your diet may also help reduce dark spots, especially due to its iron, potassium, niacin, copper and vitamin C-rich content. Consuming it as a salad or juice purifies the blood and cleanses the toxins, leaving you with healthy, glowing skin.

- **Watermelon:** Watermelon is packed with fibre and water. It contains 92 per cent water, which means it keeps your skin hydrated, soft, and supple. It also contains vitamin C, A, B1, B6, and lycopene, which are essential in improving overall skin texture. Vitamin C helps minimize the appearance of fine lines and wrinkles, while vitamins A and B help maintain an even skin texture. Lycopene prevents tissue damage in your skin by acting as a barrier against free radicals, which contribute to increased skin inflammation and promote many skin issues.

- **Green tea:** Green tea has been long known to contribute to good skin health. This is because it has antioxidants and contains catechins that protect your skin, reduce redness, improve elasticity and increase hydration. One thing to keep in mind in the case of green tea is to avoid adding milk to it, as it can reduce the effects of the antioxidants present in green tea.

- **Broccoli:** Broccoli is rich in zinc, vitamin A, and vitamin C. It contains lutein, which helps protect your skin from oxidative damage, which is the underlying reason for dry and wrinkled skin. Broccoli florets contain a compound called sulforaphane, which has anti-cancer effects, including some types of skin cancers as well. Sulforaphane also protects against sun damage and neutralizes harmful free radicals in your body.

- **Cucumber:** Cucumber majorly contains water, which keeps the skin hydrated. Cucumber's peel contains vitamin C and vitamin K, which are vital to achieving healthy, glowing skin. Studies also suggest that sea cucumbers can help reduce the appearance of fine lines, puffy eyes, and dark circles.

- **Dark chocolate**: Dark chocolate contains cocoa powder, which is high in antioxidants and thus promotes skin hydration, reduces roughness and scaliness, makes it more resistant to sunburn and improves blood flow, which brings more nutrients to your skin. However, you must make sure to choose dark chocolate with at least 70 per cent cocoa and the least amount of sugar to maximize the benefits.

- **Peach**: Peaches are rich in vitamins C, A, E and K. They also contain calcium, other minerals, and dietary fibre for a healthy digestive system. Peaches contain antioxidants that help fight free radicals in the body, UV damage and promote a healthy glow!

- **Red grapes**: Red grapes contain resveratrol, a compound that comes from their skin. Resveratrol reduces the effects of ageing and slows the production of harmful free radicals,which damage skin cells and cause signs of ageing. Also, their seed extracts have skin-rejuvenating and wound-healing properties.

- **Tomatoes**: Tomatoes are rich in lycopene. They contain antioxidants that protect the skin from UV damage and premature ageing. They also contain natural acids that regulate sebum production, making them a good option for those with oily skin types. Lastly, they contain vitamin C, which also contributes to sun protection. Relation of Macronutrients with Skin Health

(i) Relation of Macronutrients with Skin Health

Fats

Fat is an important macronutrient that plays an essential role in many aspects of human health, including skin health. There are three main categories of fats: saturated fats, unsaturated fats and trans fats.

Saturated fats

Saturated fats are saturated with hydrogen molecules and contain only single bonds between carbon molecules. Saturation of hydrogen molecules results in saturated fats being solid at room temperature.

Advantages of saturated fats:
Consuming saturated fat staves off dry skin, inflammation and premature ageing. Our cell membranes are made of about 50 per cent saturated fat, so eating the fats we're made of keeps them healthy. Not only does saturated fat keep your skin smooth and firm, it also tastes great and is easy to fit into your lifestyle.

Disadvantages of excess saturated fats:
Processed meat, cheese, butter and hydrogenated oils are all high in saturated fats. Additionally, foods that are high in saturated fat are associated with high concentrations of insulin growth factor. Insulin growth factor stimulates the production of the sex hormones that cause acne.

3 ways to include more saturated fat in your diet:

- **Incorporate animal-based foods into your diet:** If they align with your dietary preferences and needs, regularly include sources of meat, eggs, anddairy products in your meals.
- **Enjoy fatty plant foods:** Sources of saturated fat from the plant world include coconut, cocoa butter, palm oil and palm kernel oil. Dark chocolate is mostly cocoa butter, which means you can feel good about calling it a healthy food!

- **Sauté your favourite foods:** Whether it's shrimp, broccoli or shiitake, sautéing your side dishes in some butter, coconut oil or lard adds nutrition and promotes skin health.

Sources: Milk, cheese, butter, meats such as pork, beef, lamb, and poultry, coconut and palm oil

Unsaturated fats

Unsaturated fats are fatty acids in which the hydrocarbon molecules have two carbons that share a double or triple bond and are therefore not completely saturated with hydrogen atoms. Due to the decreased saturation with hydrogen bonds, the structures are weaker and are, therefore, typically liquid (oil) at room temperature.

Unsaturated fats are of two types: MUFA and PUFA.

- **Monounsaturated fatty acids** (MUFA) are healthy fat molecules with one double-bonded fatty chain acid, and the remaining carbon atoms are single-bonded. Plant oils rich in MUFA are liquid at room temperature and semi-solid or solid when chilled.

  Sources: Natural food sources abundant in MUFA are dairy products, nuts, seeds, olives and avocados, and it is the main part of the Mediterranean diet.

  Sunflower oil contains 85 per cent MUFA, while olive oil has 75 per cent and canola oil has 58 per cent. Some of the other good sources of MUFA are almond, corn, sesame, peanut, grape seed, safflower and whole grain wheat.

- **Polyunsaturated fatty acids** (PUFA) are healthy lipid molecules that have two or more carbon-carbon double bonds. Oils rich in PUFA are liquid at room temperature; viscosity and melting point temperature increase inversely to double bond.

  Sources: Good sources of PUFA are walnuts, sunflower seeds, flaxseeds and poppy seeds.

PUFAs are of two types: omega-3 fatty acids and omega-6 fatty acids.

Are you banning fat from your diet in a quest to whittle that waist? Your skin won't thank you.

Healthy bodies need healthy fats, and healthy skin needs essential fatty acids. They're called essential fatty acids (EFA) for a reason—your body needs them! It doesn't make EFAs on its own; you only get them from the foods you eat. Essential fatty acids like omega-3s and omega-6s are the building blocks of healthy cell membranes. These polyunsaturated fats also help produce the skin's natural oil barrier, which is critical in keeping skin hydrated, plumper, and younger-looking. If you're not getting enough EFAs in your diet, your skin may be dry, inflamed, and prone to whiteheads and blackheads. Yet there's more to essential fatty acids than plumper skin. EFAs can be real skincare powerhouses.

Omega fatty acids are specific types of polyunsaturated fats, which are essential additions to your diet and your skincare regime. Omega fatty acids are essential for regulating the cell membrane, helping to keep essential nutrients in the skin while expelling toxins and waste out of the skin. These are essential for maintaining radiant, healthy skin. Fatty acids work as 'building blocks' of the skin, helping to create a smooth, even-looking complexion. Omega fatty acids help to deeply hydrate the skin, helping to diminish the appearance of dry, flaky and dehydrated skin. Omega fatty acids get their names based on their molecular characteristics, and out of the eleven varieties of omega fatty acids, there are three that are the most beneficial to your skin: omega-3, omega-6, and omega-9.

- **Omega-3 fatty acids**: Omega-3 fatty acids boast anti-inflammatory benefits, helping to reduce redness, diminish the appearance of breakouts and reduce the occurrence of acne. They can regulate the skin's oil production, improve balanced hydration, subdue breakouts and minimize signs of ageing.

  Sources: Salmon, mackerel, flax, safflower oil, walnuts, sardines, soy, fortified eggs, chia seeds, hemp seeds and flaxseeds

- **Omega-6 fatty acids:** They play a vital role in regulating the normal function of the skin, helping to maintain the integrity of the skin's barrier function. The anti-inflammatory benefits of omega-6 soothe inflamed and irritated skin. Omega-6 fatty acids are known to hydrate rough skin, fade hyperpigmentation, improve wound healing and treat acne problems.

  Sources: Eggs, grapeseed oil, peanut butter, almonds, avocado, olives,whole grain foods, nuts, pumpkin seeds, pine nuts and walnuts

However, the major food sources of EPA and DHA are fish oils and krill oil.

- **Omega-9 fatty acids**: If you suffer from dry and flaky skin, omega-9 could help you as it works to maintain the level of hydration within the dermis. It has also been shown to improve the elasticity of the skin, helping to keep it looking plump and youthful. It maintains hydration, improves skin elasticity, reduces wrinkles, softens skin and reduces inflammation.

  Sources: Olive oil, almond oil, walnuts, animal fat, fish and avocado

- **Ratio: The ideal omega-3, 6 and 9 proportions are 2:1:1.**

Here are a few ideas for how to use healthy fats in your kitchen:

- **Cook with healthy oils:** Olive, canola, soy, peanut, sunflower, corn and other oils from plants are the best choices since they are high in healthy unsaturated fat. If you have a dish that requires the flavour of butter, use a very small amount of butter mixed with a neutral-flavoured oil, such as canola oil. Keep in mind that it's okay to cook with extra-virgin olive oil. The healthy fats in extra-virgin olive oil are stable at temperatures used in home cooking, with the exception of deep-fat frying or stir-frying. Then we'd advise using an oil that's more stable, like peanut oil.

- **Bake with healthy oils**: You can replace the butter in many baked goods with vegetable oils. Just cut back on the amount of oil by 25 per cent; butter contains some water, so that's why you can use less oil.

- **Serve healthy fats at the table**: Drizzle extra virgin olive oil or nut oils on vegetables instead of butter. Use peanut butter, trans fat-free margarine, or refrigerated extra virgin olive oil as a spread for whole grain toast instead of spreading on cream cheese. Pare calories by pairing healthy fats with low-calorie foods. Use oils and nuts to add flavour to lower-calorie, high-fibre foods, such as vegetables, beans, and whole grains.

- **Cut 'fast carbs' and replace them with 'slow carbs' and healthy fats.** Slow carbs include beans, non-starchy vegetables, and minimally processed whole grains, such as whole wheat berries, barley, quinoa, or brown rice. There are many delicious ways to switch from fast carbs to slow carbs. For example, instead of making white pasta or potatoes as a side dish, try making smaller portions of whole grain pasta, quinoa, or dried beans and preparing them with flavourful plant oils, nuts, and seeds.

- **Use full-fat cheese in small amounts.** Low-fat cheeses are not really that much lower in saturated fat than their full-fat counterparts, and they are often higher in sodium. A healthier strategy is to just use a small amount of full-fat, full-flavoured cheese in a dish.

- **If you're serving chicken, there's no need to strip the skin.** Chicken skin has had a bad rap for being high in fat. But most of the fat in chicken skin is healthy, unsaturated fat, and cooking with the skin keeps the chicken flavourful and moist, so you don't need to add as much salt or use a breaded coating.

(ii) Role of Ghee in Skin Health

Often called clarified butter, ghee is a golden-yellow semi-liquid with a distinct aroma and flavour. A highly-regarded ingredient in Ayurveda, or Indian traditional medicine, ghee is derived from the Sanskrit word 'ghrta'. It's believed to have originated in India and has been used since antiquity for cooking, rituals and healing. Ghee is made up of essential short-chain fatty acids as well as fat-soluble vitamins, including butyric acid and omega-3 fatty acids, arachidonic, linolenic, vitamin A, vitamin B12, vitamin D, vitamin E and vitamin K. It softens and hydrates skin, provides a natural glow, lightens dark spots, repairs dry or damaged skin,protects from cold, dry, and windy weather, treats cracked lips, reduces dark circles, rejuvenates the eyes, and heals minor wounds.

Benefits

- **Skin health**: Ghee is rich in omega fatty acids and antioxidants, and it may help neutralize free radicals and nourish the skin. It helps in the moisturization of the skin and gives it a shiny effect. Ghee helps transform dull skin into healthy skin with its nutritional benefits. It allows potent ingredients to permeate the skin and facilitates deeper absorption of herbal concentrates.

- **Skin hydration:** Since ghee contains vitamin A and rich fatty acids, it's a natural moisturizer that helps provide deep, lasting hydration.

- **Skin brightening and pigmentation**: Ghee adds glow and brightens the skin and may help activate collagen production. Ghee also has a brightening effect on the skin due to the presence of antioxidants, which may help prevent and reduce damage from oxidative stress.

- **Skin smoothing**: Ghee's beneficial ingredients can help improve skin elasticity, both by eating it and applying it to the skin. As it penetrates to the tissue level, it helps strengthen collagen and maintain elasticity.

- With ghee, the skin is held together by epidermal lipids, a type of oily wax found in the outermost layer of the dermis. These band together to prevent permeability, retain moisture and form a physical protective barrier against free radicals, oxidants, dust, bacteria and pollution at the top layer of the skin, just under the surface.

- Ghee with ceramides and fatty acids as topical ingredients can help fight dryness, fine lines and irritation.

(iii) Roles of Certain Compounds

Proteins:

- Protein is a repairing agent that provides strength, structural support and sheen to your skin. Where elastin and collagen fibres form the framework of the skin, they also contribute to keeping it healthy and firm.
- On the one hand, keratin helps to keep the skin firm, while collagen and elastin make the skin smooth while improving its elasticity.
- As we are aware of the fact that collagen production tends to decline after a certain age, which results in sagging skin, fine lines, wrinkles and other signs of ageing.
- Consuming protein in adequate amounts and making it a part of your regular diet helps boost collagen production and will retain your youthful glow for a long time while keeping signs of ageing at bay.

Fibre:

- Fibre helps to improve the circulation of blood, keeps it thin, and improves the supply of oxygen and nutrients to skin cells, thus improving your skin's appearance from the inside out. The most important thing you can do to have glowing, youthful skin is to improve your diet. For example, consume apple, avacado, papaya and guava.

Collagen builders:

- Collagen builder helps replenish vital collagen that decreases due to various factors like age, pollution or stress, making your skin healthier and more radiant. This cell-growth-stimulating property can help boost collagen production in your skin. For example, plant collagen and retinoids

Collagen supplements:

- Taking daily collagen supplements of between 2.5g and 10g shows promising results for skin ageing and could help improve skin elasticity and hydration with no adverse effects. For example, marine collagen

(iv) Relation between Antioxidants and Skin

Much like pollutants, free radicals are everywhere, but the harm they cause can be less noticeable, at least at first. At the same time, the damage they cause to your health and skin is no joke. Let's understand the flowchart below as to how antioxidants come into play for skin protection and help in healing skin.

What are free radicals?

- These are unstable molecules that can cause damage to our cells. What makes them unstable is that they are missing electrons from their outer shell. This causes them to search for other atoms or molecules that have these electrons in order for them to feel whole again and become stable.

↓

Where are free radicals present?

- Free radicals exist in our environment and can be generated from substances in the food we eat, the medicines we take, the air we breathe and the water we drink. Common causes are air pollution, sunlight (UV radiation), smoking, alcohol, pesticides and poor nutrition.

↓

Free radicals are harmful to the body and skin:

- Due to their reactive nature, free radicals can wreak havoc on your skin and other cells in their quest to find an electron and feel whole again. In order to stabilize themselves, free radicals try to bond with other atoms or molecules.

↓

This process results in oxidative stress, which can damage DNA and other parts of the cell.

↓

What is oxidative stress?

- Oxidative stress weakens living cells and tissues and can leave you more vulnerable to certain health issues. When you leave an apple or avocado on the counter, it turns brown. That is an example of oxidation or deterioration caused by free radicals.

↓

Relation with skin ageing:

- In terms of DNA, free radicals' harm done there can cause acceleration in skin ageing. External, premature ageing is the biggest threat to skin. Since our skin is our largest organ, it is also vulnerable to free radicals.

↓

How to get rid of free radicals:

- Avoiding the major free radical triggers mentioned above is a great start, but loading up on antioxidants can help.

↓

Antioxidants are compounds that can be found in food and in skincare that stop or delay damage to our cells. They work by binding to free radicals, which prevents them from binding to your healthy cells and damaging them.

↓

How to use antioxidants

- Incorporating antioxidants into your daily diet and skincare routines is pretty darn easy.
- For starters, eating a diet rich in blueberries, argan oil, green tea, dark chocolate (yes, chocolate!), and even red wine can help shield you from the negative effects of free radicals. At the same time, topical antioxidants

are sometimes better suited for preventing free radical damage to skin.

- Using serums, as they usually have a higher concentration of active ingredients and tend to penetrate more easily into the skin.

↓

When to take antioxidants

- Use them in the a.m. to prevent and in the p.m. to repair.

It is recommended that antioxidants be used only in the mornings, as they would help fight damage caused by the sun's UV rays and pollution throughout the day. But using them at night as well is a must, as it helps fight and repair the ongoing damage that was caused during the day and helps stimulate our own body's antioxidants.

CHAPTER 11

GUIDELINES FOR HEALTHY AND RADIANT SKIN

- **Consume at least five servings of fruit and vegetables each day:** Fruit and vegetables are high in antioxidants, which protect the skin from free radical damage. Wrinkling and age spots can be caused by free radicals, smoking, pollution and sunshine. Consume a rainbow of colourful fruits and vegetables on a daily basis, aiming for at least five pieces. Beta carotene, which can be found in carrots, sweet potatoes and pumpkin; and lutein, which can be found in kale, papaya and spinach, are powerful antioxidants that are essential for skincell formation and tone.

- **Eat enough vitamin C:** Vitamin C is a powerful antioxidant. It is required to maintain the immune system, produce glowing skin and aid in the healing of blemishes. Blackcurrants, blueberries, broccoli, guava, kiwi fruits, oranges, papaya, strawberries and sweet potatoes are its finest sources. Vitamin C is required for the formation of collagen, which helps strengthen the capillaries that supply the skin.

- **Avoid crash diet:** Losing and gaining weight on a regular basis might causes stretch marks on your skin. Crash diets are frequently deficient in important vitamins and minerals. This form of dieting will have an effect on your skinover time. It's always ideal to consume a well-balanced, healthy diet.

- **Stock up on selenium:** Selenium is an extremely potent antioxidant. It supports the immune system by working in conjunction with other antioxidants such as vitamins E and C. According to research, eating a selenium-rich diet can help prevent skin cancer, UV damage and age spots. Brazil nuts are one way to increase your consumption. The recommended daily quantity is provided by just four nuts (RDA). As a snack or salad garnish, combine Brazil nuts with other vitamin E-rich seeds. Fish, shellfish, eggs, wheat germ, tomatoes and broccoli are also good sources of selenium.

- **Eat enough vitamin E:** Vitamin E protects the skin from oxidative (cell) damage and promotes the formation of healthy skin. Almonds, avocados, hazelnuts, pine nuts, and sunflower and corn oils are all high in vitamin E.

- **Drink six to eight glasses of water a day:** Moisture is required for the skin to remain flexible. Your skin will appear dry, weary, and slightly grey if you are even slightly dehydrated. Drink six to eight glasses of water every day; all fluids count, but water is the best. Keep a large bottle of water on your desk if you work in an office to remind you to drink. Remember that some fruits and vegetables, such as watermelon, courgette, and cucumber, provide fluids, and the minerals they contain can help you hydrate your body and skin faster. Avoid smoking and heavy alcohol usage, as both can cause premature ageing of the skin. Hydration aids in the removal of toxins from the body and nourishes the skin. It helps in the treatment of acne, has anti-ageing properties, and keeps the skin hydrated, moist, and bright. It also aids in the maintenance of skin elasticity, making the skin appear supple, youthful and radiant.

- **Drink herbal tea:** Teas that are caffeine-free and herbal are also helpful. Herbal tea has long been used to generate a healthy glow and maintain clean and bright skin. Herbal tea stimulates metabolism and protects the skin from free radical damage. Antioxidants in herbal and green tea assist to combat the signs of ageing and keep skin moisturized.

- **Eat some healthy fat:** Essential fatty acids are found in monounsaturated and polyunsaturated fats, which can be found in avocados, oily fish, nuts, and seeds. They function as a natural moisturizer for your skin, keeping it smooth and enhancing suppleness. These fats also include a healthy dosage of vitamin E (a nutrient that many of us are deficient in), which can help protect against free radical damage.

- **Opt for omega-3:** Make sure you get enough omega-3 and omega-6 fats. These are essential fatty acids, which means they cannot be made in the body and must be obtained through the diet. You will find omega-3s in oily fish and plant sources such as linseed and its oil, chia seeds, walnuts, and rapeseed oil. Omega-3 fats encourage the body to produce anti-inflammatory compounds,which may help with inflammatory skin conditions such as eczema and psoriasis.

- **Eat more phytoestrogens:** Phytoestrogens are natural chemicals found in plant foods (phyto from the Greek word for plant). They have a similar structure to the female sex hormone oestrogen and have been found to help keep our natural hormones in balance. There are different types; some are found in soya bean products (isoflavones), such as tofu, whereas others are found in the fibre of whole grains, fruit, vegetables, and linseed (lignans). Include phyto-oestrogen-rich soya, wholegrains, fruits and vegetables as part of a balanced diet.

- **Go for low-GI carbs:** The glycaemic index (GI) is a system that ranks carbohydrate-based foods based on how slowly or quickly they are broken down in the body into glucose. Try to eat plenty of beans, pulses, porridge, and other low-GI, slow-releasing carbohydrates. These release sugar into the bloodstream gradually, providing you with a steady supply of energy and leaving you feeling satisfied for longer and therefore less likely to snack. Avoid high-GI carbohydrates like biscuits and sugary drinks, as they lead to the production of insulin, which may damage collagen and accelerate wrinkles.

- **Eat plenty of zinc:** Zinc is involved in the normal functioning of the sebaceous glands in the skin (which produce oil) and helps to repair skin damage and keep skin soft and supple. Zinc-rich foods include fish, lean red meat, wholegrains, poultry, nuts, seeds and shellfish.

CHAPTER 12

ORGANIC NATURAL INGREDIENTS FOR GLOWING SKIN

- **Lemon:** Lemons, like other citrus fruits, are natural bleaching agents. They're full of vitamin C, which promotes collagen production, making skin firmer. Lemon juice exfoliates dead skin cells and reduces the production of melanin. It has antibacterial properties that fight acne. Pure lemon juice may be too strong for most, so mix it with yoghurt and honey to make a mask. Apply this twice or thrice a week at night to reverse tanning.

- **Honey:** Honey is a wonderful ingredient as it is a natural bleaching agent, moisturizing and antibacterial. It helps even skin tone and prevents acne. You can put raw honey directly on the face or mix it in masks to get clear, glowing skin.

- **Papaya:** Papaya has papain that increases cell turnover, revealing brighter skin from within. The alpha-hydroxy acids found in papaya make it one of the best home remedies for pimple marks. You can mash a few pieces into a smooth paste and apply it where needed. Leave it for 20 minutes before you wash it with lukewarm water.

- **Yoghurt:** Yoghurt has lactic acid, one of the mildest AHAs, and is suitable for sensitive skin. It gently exfoliates and works as a melanin suppressor. Regular application of yoghurt can reduce the appearance of blemishes and enhance your skin tone. Apply it directly or mix it into a mask for softness and glow.

- **Licorice:** Licorice root extracts have glabridin, which inhibits tyrosinase, a melanin-producing enzyme. It has liquiritin, which breaks melanin and removes pigmentation, making your skin look clearer. It is great for removing acne scars and soothing irritated skin.

- **Turmeric:** Turmeric has antibacterial, anti-inflammatory and antioxidant properties, making it effective for acne-prone skin. Curcumin, present in turmeric, suppresses melanin production and instantly lightens skin tone. A popular brightening ingredient, turmeric treats various skin issues besides providing essential nutrients. You can mix half a teaspoon of turmeric into any mask to get a glow.

- **Potato:** Potatoes are packed with vitamin B6 and effectively exfoliate and lighten skin tone. If you are wondering how to remove spots from the face, make a potato paste or extract the juice and mix it with honey, lemon or rose water to make a mask. It is very useful for removing dark circles.

- **Gram Flour**: Gram flour is an extremely safe yet effective, nutrient-rich skin brightener. It contains beta-carotene, niacin, riboflavin, folate acid and unsaturated fatty acids that moisturize skin while removing excess oil. It can be used as a gentle everyday cleanser by rubbing a small amount with water or rose water like a scrub. It exfoliates dead skin cells to reveal soft, healthy skin, bringing out a natural glow.

- **Aloe vera:** Aloe vera is one of the mildest natural bleaching agents and is ideal for people with sensitive skin to lighten the complexion. It has a compound called 'anthraquinone' that gently exfoliates dead skin. It also contains 'lignin', which improves skin's elasticity, and antioxidants that fight pollution and sun damage. Apply aloe vera gel directly to clean skin or mix it with honey to make a mask or with brown sugar to make a brightening scrub.

- **Neem:** Neem has antibacterial and antifungal properties that would keep acne at bay, which in turn would prevent the formation of acne marks. It also has cooling properties that would reduce redness, dark spots, and blemishes and purify pollutants from pores to reveal even, glowing skin. Applying a neem and sandalwood mask can tighten skin and reduce signs of ageing, making your skin glow naturally.

- **Oats:** Oats, known as a superfood, are excellent for the skin due to their cleansing, exfoliating and many other benefits. It has 'saponin', which flushes skin-dulling toxins, and antioxidants that boost skin's health to promote a natural glow. It also contains amino acids, vitamin B1, zinc, etc., that reverse discolouration and the appearance of dark spots. Use oat milk or ground oats with honey and milk to make a brightening mask. All of the above ingredients are safe and effective methods for lightening skin without any side effects.

CHAPTER 13

SKINCARE ROUTINE

Great skin is not simply a matter of DNA—your daily habits, in fact, have a big impact on what you see in the mirror. But depending on which product reviews you read or which doctors you consult, there are a dizzying number of opinions on everything from how to moisturize to how to protect yourself from UV rays. Ultimately, caring for your skin is simply personal. Here's what you should keep in mind to sort through all the noise:

The three main steps of skincare are the following:

(i) Cleansing

Wash twice a day, morning and night, to avoid clogged pores, dullness and acne. Find your facial cleanser. The right formula cleanses your skin without stripping it of essential, healthy oils. Take it easy with exfoliating scrubs (use once a week) and avoid those with crushed walnut shells or abrasive ingredients.

(ii) Toning

Toners should be applied after cleansing and before putting on anything else. The traditional application method is to saturate a cotton pad and pass it over your face.

Tip: Applying toner with clean hands is the most efficient. Just pour a few drops into your palm, then swipe it on. If you prefer, you can pull apart a cotton pad so it's not so thick before putting toner on it. Most formulas can be used morning and night, but you might want to use those with exfoliating acids only at night or every other day. Here are some hero ingredients to look for:

- → Alpha and beta hydroxy acids gently remove dead skin cells that can clog pores, improve sun-damaged skin and minimize dullness.
- → Hyaluronic acid boosts hydration, seals in dewiness and plumps skin to subtly treat fine lines.
- → Rose water and green tea calm irritation and reduce redness with an anti-inflammatory effect.
- → Vitamin E and C fight daily exposure to free radicals that can age your skin.

(III) Treating with Serums

Serums are powerful skin allies. Filled with concentrated doses of active ingredients, these elixirs can mitigate a number of issues, from dark spots to wrinkles.

→ Hyaluronic acid helps seal in hydration and strengthen the barrier function (the top layer of your skin) to prevent moisture loss.

→ Vitamin C brightens dull skin and decreases dark spots with continued use.

→ Retinol, vitamin B3 and peptides stimulate the production of collagen and elastin, proteins in the body that help prevent lines and skin sagging.

→ Colloidal sulfur and niacinamide calm redness and irritation by decreasing inflammation, preventing acne with their antimicrobial effects.

(iv) Moisturizing

The most basic function of a moisturizer is to hydrate and soften the skin. Essentially, moisturizers assist in preventing water loss through the outer layers of the skin.

(v) Completing with Sunscreen

Sunscreen is, hands down, the most crucial skincare product. It's of utmost importance as part of your year-round regimen, and consistent sunscreen use helps to prevent the development of fine lines and wrinkles, textural imperfections, and changes in the appearance of pores over time. More importantly, daily sunscreen use can help prevent the formation of certain skin cancers.

CHAPTER 14

HEALTHY SKIN HABITS

Your skin is a natural barrier against abrasion, chemicals and infections. The best approach to maintaining healthy skin is to practise proper skin hygiene. Next, we understand how different factors act as support for the skin's glow:

(i) Skin Hygiene

Importance of Skin Hygiene

→ The stratum corneum layer and its protective barrier function require both moisture (hydration) and lipids (fats and oils).

→ Skin also requires a diverse population of indigenous microorganisms to protect it from disease-causing infections. Excessively severe and frequent skin washing can wipe away the native germs, allowing disease-causing microbes to thrive.

Steps for Cleaning Skin

- Wash with mild soaps and cleansers to remove daily filth and grime. Hands should be washed for at least ten to fifteen seconds to be effective. Scrubbing with abrasive materials should be avoided.
- Look for skin cleansers that have mild-surface active agents, as well as moisturizers and emollients that are not too acidic or alkaline. Avoid using harsh soaps and detergents on your skin since they can peel away protective layers and eliminate skin oils and lipids.
- Wash your hands with lukewarm water. Using hot water can cause skin to become overly dry and damaged.
- After washing, make sure to thoroughly cleanse your skin.
- Thoroughly dry your hands and skin. Do not rub the skin while it dries.
- Carefully choose skincare products. Fragrances and preservatives in many over-the-counter lotions and creams might irritate your skin.

(ii) Workout

Working out tones the skin, increases blood circulation, and oxygenates it, giving it a healthy glow.

- Exercise results in the production of sweat. Sweat clears pores by removing dead skin cells, oils, and pollutants that accumulate over time.

- Workout can assist in giving oxygen and nutrients to the skin by increasing heart rate and enhancing blood circulation, which maintains the skin healthy, increases collagen formation, and encourages new skin cells, which keeps the skin looking beautiful and is also beneficial for anti-ageing.

(iii) Yoga for Face

- **Puffing the cheek:** In this face yoga for glowing skin, you should inhale deeply and then distend the air from cheek to cheek till they are completely puffed out, and then release the air. This exercise will make the cheek muscles strong and make them look full. This exercise, if done regularly, will lift and plump the cheeks.
- **Chanting Om with a smile:** Few people are unaware of the benefits of chanting OM because it relaxes both the mind and the facial muscles. This yoga for face skin tightening is the easiest facial yoga exercise. Close your eyes and bring a slight smile to your face, with your focus on the point between the eyebrows. Most people have the habit of frowning without realizing it, and this can form wrinkles. However, doing this facial yoga of chanting OM will offset the wrinkles and provide the skin with a tightening effect.
- **Lifting the eyebrows:** In this face yoga for a glowing face, you need to place the first finger of your hand around half an inch above your eyebrows and lift the eyebrows while pushing them down with the finger.

Repeat this exercise ten to twelve times during the day. The forehead is the first part of the face to develop wrinkles. With this exercise, the muscles and skin of the forehead will be tightened, and the skin will glow.

→ **Making a face like a fish:** Pull in the insides of your cheeks like you're making the face of a fish. Hold this position in the yoga exercise for a face glow while you keep your eyes open. You should keep this pose until your eyes start to water. You then blink and release the pose. This is a great exercise for the cheeks, which will look youthful, supple, and flushed. Usually, the skin of the cheeks sags fast, and the exercise prevents that from happening.

→ **Smile and pout:** This yoga for face glow improves the downward drift and makes your jawline and cheeks flushed. For this exercise, you need to push the lips out as much as possible as if you are going to kiss and then smile broadly. You should repeat this exercise fifteen times a day. This exercise enhances the youthfulness of the chin and cheeks together.

(iv) Stress

Sleep deprivation causes stress, which promotes indications of ageing like fine wrinkles, elasticity loss, and uneven pigmentation, according to research. When you don't get enough sleep, stress can lead to hyperpigmentation, early ageing, patchy and uneven skin tone, dry skin, acne, and dark circles. Redness, inflamed skin, severe dryness, dehydrated skin, irritation and itchiness, stinging or burning sensations while applying products, increased breakouts, and overall dullness of the face are all indicators of a strained skin barrier.

Excess cortisol, for example, can hasten the breakdown of collagen and elastin, the proteins that give skin its youthful texture. Cortisol causes your skin glands to produce more oil, which can block pores and trigger acne breakouts. Chronic stress causes constant increases in these hormones, which can be harmful to your skin's health.

→ **Take several deep breaths:** This makes you breathe more slowly and allows your muscles to relax. The extra oxygen tells your brain to slow down and relax your body.

→ **Stretch:** Stretching can also help you relax and feel less tense by allowing your muscles to relax.

→ **Make a list of your ideas:** Keeping a gratitude notebook or simply writing down the things for which you are grateful might help you cope with stress.

→ **Dedicate some time to yourself:** It could be anything as simple as listening to music, reading a nice book or seeing a movie.

→ **Meditate:** Meditation, defined as a period of silence during which the mind is focused on a positive or neutral idea, has been shown in studies to reduce stress.

→ **Get plenty of rest:** To feel rested, most individuals require seven to nine hours of sleep per night.

- → **Eat healthily:** Caffeine or high-sugar snack foods provide short bursts of energy that rapidly wear off. Bananas, seafood, avocados, chicken, and dark green, leafy vegetables are good sources of B vitamins. B vitamins have been shown in studies to help reduce stress by regulating nerves and brain cells.
- → **Get up and about:** Physical activity can help you relax your muscles while also boosting your mood. Physical activity raises your body's levels of endorphins, which are 'feel-good' compounds. Endorphins can make you feel better.

(v) Skin Glow Packs

- → **Turmeric:** Mix about half a teaspoon of turmeric powder with a cup of gram flour (chickpea flour). Add milk/ water and mix well to form a smooth paste. Now, add a few drops of rose water and mix again. Apply this paste on your face and neck and leave it on till it dries. Then, rinse with cool water.
- → **Honey:** You can directly apply honey to your face and neck area, but ensure that your skin is clean and damp. Massage for a few minutes, allowing it to get absorbed by the skin. Now, wash off with lukewarm water.
- → **Milk:** You can apply raw milk to your skin or mix it with any other ingredients and form a paste. Allow it to dry and then rinse it with water.
- → **Besan:** Besan is used by mixing it with milk, water, or

any other ingredients. It is applied like a pack on the skin. Sometimes, sugar is also added to help in exfoliation.

→ **Cucumber:** Put the slices of cucumber on your eyes as they show in all the magazines and televisions. You can also put the cucumber in a mixer grinder and apply the juice.

→ **Papaya:** Papaya can be applied generously on the skin, let it dry and then rinse with tap water.

→ **Aloe vera:** Gently scrape out aloe vera gel from the leaves and apply on your skin. Leave it for ten to fifteen minutes. Then rinse your skin with cool water and pat dry.

→ **Yoghurt:** Consuming yoghurt is good for our skin. You can apply it directly on the skin using cotton, leave for ten to fifteen minutes and then wash with cold water.

→ **Banana:** Mash a banana, apply it on your skin, and leave for fifteen to twenty minutes. Then wash with lukewarm water. You can also make a facemask using one ripe banana, one tablespoon of honey and lemon juice. Banana peels also help in lightening our skin and dark circles. Gently rub banana peels on your skin. Leave for ten to fifteen minutes and then wash with water.

→ **Coconut oil:** It is rich in antioxidants and fatty acids. It reduces inflammation and does wonders for almost all skin types. It is an excellent moisturizer, cleanser and sunscreen. It keeps our skin acne free. Regular massage with lukewarm coconut oil keeps our skin glowing and healthy.

CHAPTER 15

RECIPES

The best way to get the glow you want is by taking action. You can't rely on products alone, and it's important to work with a professional who can guide you through your skincare routine. The most important thing is to understand what your skin needs and when it needs it. Here are some special recipes for skin health for you to check out:

RECIPES FOR GLOWING SKIN

Smoothies and Drinks

Beauty Water	
Ingredients	**Method**
• 5 strawberries • 1 orange, juiced • ½ lemon, juiced • 1 cup coconut water • 5 mint leaves	• Purée the strawberries in a blender, then pour into a glass. • Add in the rest of the ingredients into this glass. • Garnish the water with mint leaves, and your done making it.

Turmeric Ginger Power Drink	
Ingredients	**Method**
• 10 g turmeric powder • 50 g fresh ginger • 2 lemons, juiced • 1 glass water	• Wash the ginger and peel it. • Place all ingredients in a blender and blend until smooth. • Strain and enjoy.

Orange Carrot Smoothie	
Ingredients	**Method**
• ½ cup orange • ½ cup carrot • ½ tsp cinnamon powder • 1 inch ginger • 1 cup water	• Place all the ingredients in the mixer grinder. • Blend until smooth. • Pour into the glass. • Serve it.

ABC Smoothie (Apple, Beetroot, Carrot)	
Ingredients	**Method**
• ½ cup apple • ½ cup beetroot • ½ cup carrot • ¼ tsp cinnamon • 1 inch ginger • 4–5 basil leaves • 1 cup water	• Place all the ingredients in the mixer grinder. • Blend it until smooth. • Pour it into the glass. • Serve it.

Cucumber Pear Juice	
Ingredients	**Method**
• 1 small cucumber • 1 small pear • 6–8 mint leaves • 4–6 basil leaves • ½ lemon, juiced • Rock salt as per the taste • 1 cup water	• Mix all the ingredients in the mixer grinder. • Blend it until smooth. • Pour it into the glass. • Serve it and enjoy.

Amla Aloe Vera Drink	
Ingredients	**Method**
• ½ cup amla • 2 tbsp aloe vera juice • ½ tsp cumin powder • Rock salt as per the taste	• Place all the ingredients in the mixer grinder. • Blend it until smooth. • Pour it in the glass. • Serve and enjoy.

Red Smoothie	
Ingredients	**Method**
• 1 ripe banana • ½ cup cucumber • 1 spinach • 2 broccoli • 4 strawberries • 1 beetroot • ½ lemon	• Add all the ingredients to a blender. • Blend it until smooth. • Add ice (optional). • Serve chilled.

Red Smoothie	
Ingredients	**Method**
• ½ cup tender coconut water • 1 tsp flaxseed powder • 2 almonds • 2 tbsp coconut cream	

Strawberry Smoothie	
Ingredients	**Method**
• 3 fresh figs • 3 strawberries • 1 banana • 2 cups of any plant-based • Honey as per taste	• Combine all the ingredients and place it in a blender. • Blend it • Add ice (optional). • Serve chilled.

Walnut Banana Smoothie	
Ingredients	**Method**
• 2 ripe bananas • 2–4 walnuts • 1 tbsp of chia seeds • 2 cups of plant-based milk	• Combine all the ingredients and place it in a blender. • Blend it until smooth. • Add ice (optional). • Serve chilled.

Blueberry Smoothie	
Ingredients	**Method**
• Blueberry: 1 cup (fresh or frozen) • 1 banana • 1 tsp chia seeds • 1 cup tender coconut water • ½ cup almonds • 1 tsp honey	• Add all the ingredients to a blender. • Blend it until smooth. • Add ice (optional). • Serve chilled.

Soup Recipes

Pumpkin Soup	
Ingredients	**Method**
• 2 cups or 250 g pumpkin • 1 medium or ⅓ cup onion, chopped • 1-2 small garlic cloves, roughly chopped • 1 cup water • 2 tsp olive oil (optional) • ¼ tsp dry oregano • ½ tsp dry thyme • Crushed pepper powder as required	• Rinse, peel, and chop pumpkin in cubes. Also, onion and garlic cloves. • Add the pumpkin cubes, chopped onions and garlic to a pressure cooker. • Now add 1 cup of water. For a thicker soup, add less water. • Cover and pressure cook on medium heat for 8 to 9 minutes.

Pumpkin Soup	
Ingredients	**Method**
• Salt as required **For garnishing:** 1 to 2 tbsp bread croutons (optional) 1 tbsp whipping cream (optional)	If you do not have a pressure cooker, you can even cook the pumpkin cubes in a pan. Add water as required if cooking in a pan. • When the pressure settles down, open the lid. Let the pumpkin mixture become warm. • Then, with the hand-held mixer or beater, blend the whole mixture. You can even add the mixture to a blender or grinder jar, and then blend it to a smooth purée. Do not blend when hot, as then the mixture splutters. • Blend till smooth. You can keep the soup slightly chunky if you want. • Now keep the cooker back on the stovetop on a low to medium flame. Add olive oil.

Pumpkin Soup	
Ingredients	**Method**
	• Adding olive oil is optional, and you can skip it completely. You can even add coconut oil or sunflower oil instead of olive oil. • Mix very well. • Then add oregano, thyme and crushed black pepper as required. • Add sugar (optional) and salt as per taste. • Mix well. If the pumpkin is sweet, then skip adding sugar. • Let the soup come to a gentle simmer until it becomes hot. Then switch off the flame. • Serve pumpkin soup hot or warm. You can garnish with some grated cheese, herbs, bread croutons or cream. This soup can be served chilled too.

Lemon Coriander Soup Serves 2	
Ingredients	**Method**
• 1 tbsp ghee or cold pressed coconut oil or olive oil • 1 tsp finely chopped ginger or 1-inch ginger • 1 tsp finely chopped garlic or 3 to 4 medium garlic cloves • 1/4 cup chopped spring onion whites, 2 small spring onions, or 1/4 cup finely chopped onions • 1/4 to 1/3 cup finely chopped carrots or 1 small to medium carrot • 1 to 1.25 cups chopped mushrooms or 4 to 5 white button mushrooms • 1 green chilli (chopped)	• Heat 1 tbsp of ghee or cold-pressed coconut oil or olive oil in a large pot over medium heat. • Add 1 tsp of finely chopped ginger and 1 tsp of finely chopped garlic to the pot. Sauté for about 1 minute until fragrant. • Add ¼ cup of chopped spring onion whites (or 2 small spring onions, or ¼ cup finely chopped onions) and ¼ to ⅓ cup of finely chopped carrots (or 1 small to medium carrot). Sauté for another 2–3 minutes until the vegetables start to soften. • Next, add 1 to 1.25 cups of chopped mushrooms (or 4 to 5 white button mushrooms) and 1 chopped green chili. Cook for an additional 2–3 minutes until the mushrooms are tender.

Lemon Coriander Soup Serves 2	
Ingredients	**Method**
• 1 lemongrass stalk (optional) • Crushed black pepper or black pepper powder as required • Salt as required • 4 cups of water • 2 tbsp lemon juice or add as per taste • 1⁄3 cup chopped coriander leaves • 1 to 2 tbsp chopped spring onion greens • Scallions (optional) **For garnishing:** • 1 tbsp coriander leaves • 4 lemon slices (optional) • 1 tbsp chopped spring onion greens (scallions) or chives (optional)	• If using, add 1 lemongrass stalk (optional) for additional flavour. • Season the soup with crushed black pepper or black pepper powder and salt according to your taste preferences. • Pour in 4 cups of water and bring the soup to a boil. Reduce the heat to low and let it simmer for 10-15 minutes to allow the flavours to meld together. • Stir in 2 tbsp of lemon juice (adjust to taste) and ⅓ cup of chopped coriander leaves. Cook for another 1-2 minutes. • Serve the soup hot, garnished with additional chopped coriander leaves, lemon slices (optional), and chopped spring onion greens (scallions) or chives (optional).

Bean Tomato Soup	
Ingredients	**Method**
• ½ cup onion • ½ cup tomato • 50 g coriander leaves • 4 garlic cloves • 1 cup vegetable broth • 200 g cooked kidney beans • 1 tsp salt • 1 tsp black pepper • 2 tbsp peanut butter • 5 mint leaves	• Sauté coriander leaves, tomato and onion till the onion turns translucent. • Add garlic and cook for one to two minutes. • After two minutes, add the cooked beans and vegetable broth. • Put the mixture in a blender and add peanut butter. • After this, use salt and pepper to season this mixture in a pan. • Serve this soup with mint leaves.

Walnut Beet Soup	
Ingredients	**Method**
• ½ cup walnuts • 2 tsp oil • 1 bay leaf • 1 small onion • 4 cloves of garlic • 1 green chilli • ½ tsp ginger	• Blend all the ingredients in a blender. • Remove the mixture from the blender until the consistency is smooth. • Take the mixture to a pot, and heat it on a low flame, and season it.

Walnut Beet Soup	
Ingredients	**Method**
• 1 large beetroot • 2 cup vegetable stock • 2 tsp salt • 2 tsp pepper • ¼ cup coconut milk • 10 g coriander leaves	• Stir the soup and add coriander for garnishing, and enjoy.

Tomato Cashew Nut Soup	
Ingredients	**Method**
• 2 cups of tomato • 1 onion • 4 cloves of garlic • 2 tbsp salt • 1 tsp black pepper • 2 tsp olive oil • 2 cups vegetable broth • ½ cup cashew nuts • 5 leaves of mint	• Sauté all the ingredients except the vegetable broth. • Blend this mix along with vegetable broth to a smooth liquid consistency. • Serve the soup with mint leaves and enjoy.

Salad Recipes

Moong Sprouts Corn salad	
Ingredients	**Method**
• 400 g corn cobs or 2 medium corn cobs • 1 small or ¼ cup onion, finely chopped • 1 small to medium or ⅓ to ½ cup cucumber, finely chopped • 1/4 tsp red chilli powder • 1/4 tsp roasted cumin powder • 1 tbsp chopped coriander leaves • ½ to 1 tbsp lemon juice; add as per taste • Salt as required	• First steam or boil 2 medium-sized corn cobs till the kernels are tender. You can steam them in a pressure cooker or steamer. • Add the corn cobs and water to a pan. • Cover and cook till the corn kernels become tender. Add more water if required while cooking. • Add the corn kernels to a mixing bowl. • Add ¼ cup finely chopped onion, ⅓ to ½ cup finely chopped cucumber and 1 tbsp chopped coriander. • Sprinkle ¼ tsp red chilli powder and ¼ tsp roasted cumin powder. • Now add ½ to 1 tsp lemon juice. Add lemon juice as per your taste preferences. • Toss and mix everything very well. • Serve sweet corn salad.

Vegetable Salad with Nuts	
Ingredients	**Method**
• 2 medium carrots • 2 medium cucumbers • 1 large tomato • 2 to 3 spring onions • 1 or 2 tbsp pumpkin seeds • 1 tbsp roasted sunflower seeds • ½ tbsp sesame seeds • 1 tbsp chopped cashews or whole cashews • 1 tbsp chopped almonds (optional) • 1 tbsp chopped pistachios • 1 tbsp walnuts • ½ or 1 tbsp extra-virgin olive oil or cold-pressed coconut oil • ½ or 1 tsp lemon juice • 3 to 4 fresh basil • Chopped herbs as required • 1 tsp coriander, finely chopped • Salt as required • Pepper as required	• Firstly, rinse all the veggies. Peel and chop the carrots, radish and cucumber. • Chop the tomatoes. Finely chop the spring onions. Take all the veggies in a bowl. • Heat a pan and dry roast all the seeds and nuts till crisp and lightly browned. Keep it aside. • In a small bowl, whisk all the ingredients well for the dressing. Pour the dressing into the bowl containing the vegetables. • Toss well so that the veggies are coated with the dressing. Sprinkle the roasted seeds and dry fruits. • Serve the vegetable salad.

Sweet Potato Tofu Salad	
Ingredients	**Method**
• 100 g sweet potato • 1 tbsp olive oil • 1 tsp chilli flakes • 70 g tofu • 2 tbsp soy sauce • 200 g fresh spinach • 75 g green mong, steamed • 75 g tomatoes • 1 onion, sliced • 1 tsp flax seeds **For dressing:** • 2 cloves of garlic • 1 tbsp peanut butter • 1 tbsp curd • 4 tbsp lemon juice • 1 tsp salt • 1 tsp pepper	• Sauté tofu, green moong and spinach in a non-stick pan. • Boil the sweet potato, peel and cut it into cubes, and steam it. Add chilli flakes and olive oil before tossing. • Put lentils, sweet potatoes, tofu, onions and cherry tomatoes in serving-size dishes. • In a small dish, combine all the ingredients to make the dressing. • Add flax seeds, and enjoy adding the dressing to the salad bowl.

Snacks Recipes

Berries Bowl	
Ingredients	**Method**
For the smoothie portion: • 28 gm unsweetened almond milk • 1 banana • 1 cup strawberries • 1 cup frozen blueberries • Berries **For the topping:** • Sliced bananas • Sliced strawberries • Sliced kiwi • Frozen blueberries • Granola • Sliced almonds • Coconut chips • Honey (omit for vegan option)	• Run smoothie packs under hot water for 5 seconds. • Load all smoothie ingredients into the blender in the order listed and blend until smooth. (If you don't have a super blender, you may have to pause a couple times to stir in any large frozen chunks before blending again.) • Divide smoothie between two bowls, or enjoy as a smoothie, and top accordingly.

<table>
<tr><th colspan="2">Paneer Shawarma</th></tr>
<tr><th>Ingredients</th><th>Method</th></tr>
<tr><td>• 250 gm paneer
• 2 ragi rotis (refer to the recipe from Nutracy Lifestyle app)
• ½ tsp cumin powder
• ½ tsp coriander powder
• ½ tsp garam masala
• Salt to taste
• ½ tsp red chilli powder
• 2 tbsp
• 1 chopped onion
• 1 tomato, sliced
• 1 lettuce leaf</td><td>• Use a potato masher to smash the paneer.
• After that, incorporate all of the dry seasonings listed in the ingredient list.
• Heat a grill pan in the meantime, add the mixture, and cook it on both sides until the grill mark shows on both.
• Take it out and wait for 5–8 minutes.
• After making chapatis with ragi flour and properly cooking them on a tawa, add the paneer mixture.
• Spread it out.
• Add in lettuce leaf, tomato slices and onion slices for extra flavour.
• Now serve it with mint chutney on the side.</td></tr>
</table>

CHAPTER 16

THE ACTION PLAN FOR A GLOWING SKIN

ACTION 1: AFFIRMATIONS

What are affirmations?

Affirmations are like little pep talks you give yourself to boost your mindset and promote positive beliefs and behaviours. When it comes to skin health, affirmations can play a powerful role in improving your overall well-being and taking care of your skin.

Why practise affirmations for skin health?

1. **Boosts your confidence:** Affirmations can help you feel more confident in your own skin by cultivating positive thoughts and attitudes towards your skin's health and appearance.
2. **Mind-body connection:** Affirmations reinforce the connection between your mind and body, encouraging

you to prioritize self-care and adopt a holistic approach to skincare.

3. **Less stress:** Affirmations can be a great stress-reliever, and we all know that stress can wreak havoc on your skin. By reducing stress, you're giving your skin a better chance to thrive.
4. **Stay committed:** Consistency is key when it comes to skincare. Affirmations help you stay motivated and committed to your skincare routine, leading to long-term improvements.

How do affirmations help with improving skin issues?

1. **Balance from within:** Positive affirmations can help restore balance by reducing stress-induced skin issues like acne, eczema, or psoriasis.
2. **Show yourself some love:** Affirmations encourage self-care practices such as regular cleansing, moisturizing and protecting your skin, which can lead to improved skin health.
3. **Confidence is key:** Positive affirmations boost your self-confidence, reducing self-criticism and promoting self-love, which aids in the healing process of skin issues.
4. **Healthy habits, happy skin:** Affirmations reinforce positive beliefs and encourage healthy lifestyle habits, like eating a balanced diet, staying hydrated, and avoiding harmful skincare practices.

The Science Behind It:

While affirmations may seem simple, they have a scientific basis that supports their effectiveness in improving skin health:

1. **Neuroplasticity:** Repeating positive affirmations can rewire your brain, creating new neural pathways that support positive beliefs and behaviours, including better skin health.
2. **Mind–body connection:** The mind and body are intertwined, and positive affirmations can reduce stress hormones, promote relaxation, and create a more favourable environment for healthy skin.
3. **Stress reduction:** Chronic stress can lead to skin issues. Affirmations can help reduce stress levels, giving your skin a chance to heal and thrive.
4. **Placebo effect:** Believing in positive outcomes can trigger the placebo effect, influencing physiological responses and potentially improving skin conditions.
5. **Self-care and healthy habits:** Affirmations promote self-care practices and healthy habits, such as adopting a consistent skincare routine, nourishing your body with nutritious foods, staying hydrated, and protecting your skin from environmental factors.

Remember, affirmations work best when integrated into your daily routine alongside proper skincare practices and seeking professional advice when needed.

Here are some affirmations you should practise in your daily routine. Take a break. Relax.

Say these affirmations out loud, or you can write them down too.

1. 'My skin is a reflection of my overall well-being, and I'm committed to taking care of it.'

   ___

2. 'I embrace my skin's uniqueness and appreciate its beauty.'

   ___

3. 'Every day, my skin is getting healthier and more radiant.'

   ___

4. 'I am grateful for my skin and treat it with kindness and respect.'

   ___

5. 'I choose to focus on the positive aspects of my skin and let go of any negativity.'

   ___

6. 'I am confident and comfortable in my own skin, no matter what.'

   ___

7. 'I prioritize self-care, knowing that it contributes to the health and vitality of my skin.'

   ___

8. 'I release stress and tension, allowing my skin to relax and rejuvenate.'

   ___

9. 'I am patient with my skin's journey, trusting that it knows how to heal itself.'

____

10. 'I create a peaceful environment for my skin to thrive, both internally and externally.'

____

11. 'I am mindful of the products I use, opting for those that nourish and support my skin's health.'

____

12. 'I make time for self-care rituals that make my skin feel loved and pampered.'

____

13. 'I radiate confidence and positivity, which reflects in the appearance of my skin.'

____

14. 'I prioritize a healthy lifestyle, knowing it contributes to my skin's natural glow.'

____

15. 'I appreciate my skin's resilience and its ability to regenerate and renew.'

____

Action 2: Exercises

Exercise plays a vital role in promoting healthy skin. When you get moving, it improves blood circulation, delivering essential nutrients and oxygen to your skin cells. This nourishment enhances cell regeneration and gives your skin a healthy glow.

Here is how you can know if you are doing the right exercises for healthy skin:

- ☐ Post-exercise glow: Do you notice a natural, healthy glow on your skin after your workout?
- ☐ Improved complexion: Have you observed improvements in your skin's overall complexion, such as a more even tone and reduced blemishes?
- ☐ Increased skin elasticity: Does your skin appear firmer and tighter, indicating improved skin elasticity?
- ☐ Reduced stress-related skin issues: Are you experiencing fewer stress-related skin problems, such as acne breakouts or flare-ups of conditions like eczema or psoriasis?
- ☐ Enhanced skin hydration: Is your skin more hydrated, with a softer and more supple texture?
- ☐ Well-rested appearance: Do you wake up with a well-rested and rejuvenated look, indicating better sleep quality?
- ☐ Balanced exercise routine: Are you engaging in a variety of exercises, including cardiovascular workouts, strength training and flexibility exercises?
- ☐ Consistency: Are you consistently following your exercise routine to maximize the benefits for your skin?
- ☐ Sun protection: Do you take appropriate measures to protect your skin from the sun during outdoor activities, such as wearing sunscreen and protective clothing?

- ☐ Overall well-being: Are you experiencing improved overall well-being, including reduced stress levels, increased energy and a better mood?

If you're not seeing the desired results for your skin from your current exercise routine, it might be beneficial to try incorporating the following exercises. Here are some examples along with explanations of how they can potentially benefit your skin:

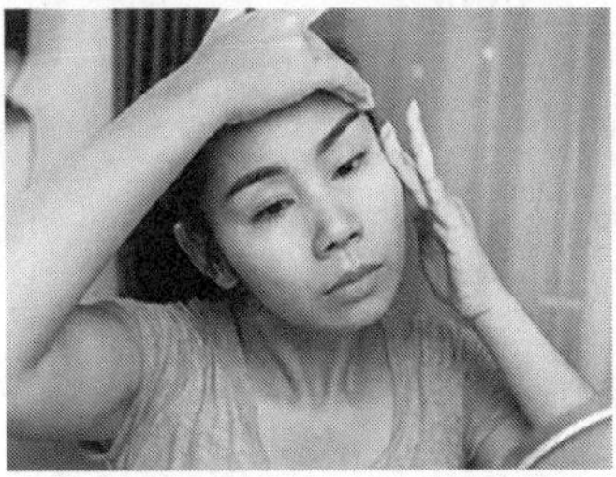

WHAT CAN YOU DO?

Exercise 1: Facial Yoga

Facial yoga involves simple exercises that target the muscles in your face, like smiling widely, puckering your lips, or raising your eyebrows. By doing these movements regularly, you can improve muscle tone and achieve a more lifted and toned appearance. Facial yoga also helps increase blood flow to your face, stimulates collagen production, and reduces the appearance of wrinkles.

***Cheek Lifter*:** Smile as wide as you can, making sure to engage your cheek muscles. Place your fingers on the top part of your

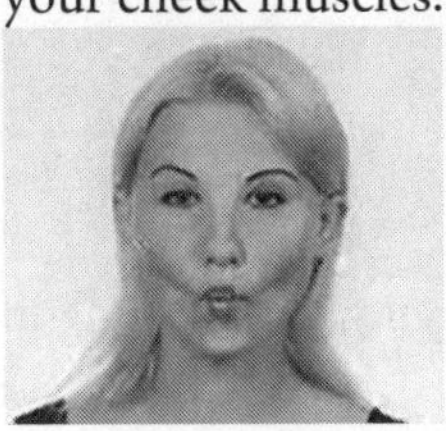

cheeks and apply a slight resistance as you try to lift your cheeks even higher. Hold for a few seconds, and then relax. Repeat several times.

Fish Face: Suck in your cheeks and lips to create a fish face or kissy face shape. Hold this position for a few seconds, feeling the muscles in your cheeks and lips contract. Relax and repeat multiple times.

Forehead Smoother: Sit with a straight back, place palms on forehead, and slide outward towards temples, smoothing wrinkles. Repeat 5–7 times for a relaxed, smoother forehead. Include this in your daily skincare routine.

Exercise 2: High-Intensity Interval Training

High-Intensity Interval Training, or HIIT, workouts are a form of exercise that involves short bursts of intense exercises followed by periods of rest or lower-intensity exercises. The idea is to push yourself hard during the intense intervals and then give yourself some recovery time before repeating the cycle.

HIIT workouts are all about quick bursts of intense exercises followed by short recovery periods. This type of workout is great for improving cardiovascular fitness, boosting blood circulation and making you sweat. By engaging in HIIT, you promote detoxification, increase oxygen supply to your skin and support a healthy complexion.

Here's a sample HIIT workout routine that focuses on promoting skin glow:

1. Warm-Up:

- ☐ Start with three minutes of light jogging or marching in place to raise your heart rate.

- ☐ Followed by dynamic stretches, such as arm circles, leg swings, and torso twists, to warm-up your muscles.

2. **Circuit 1: Perform each exercise for forty seconds, followed by a twenty-second rest. Complete three rounds:**

- ☐ Jumping Jacks: Start with your feet together and arms by your sides. Jump your feet out wide while raising your arms overhead.
- ☐ High Knees: Run in place, lifting your knees as high as possible with each step.
- ☐ Skaters: Start by jumping to the right, landing on your right foot, while sweeping your left foot behind your right leg. Repeat on the other side.

3. **Circuit 2: Perform each exercise for forty seconds, followed by a twenty-second rest. Complete three rounds:**

- ☐ Burpees: Begin in a standing position, lower into a squat, place your hands on the floor, jump your feet back into a plank position, do a push-up, jump your feet forward, and explosively jump up.
- ☐ Mountain Climbers: Get into a push-up position and quickly alternate, bringing your knees towards your chest as if running in place.

- ☐ Plank Jacks: Start in a plank position, then jump your feet wide apart and back together while maintaining a strong core.

4. **Circuit 3: Perform each exercise for forty seconds, followed by a twenty-second rest. Complete three rounds:**

- ☐ Squat Jumps: Begin in a squat position, then explode upward, jumping as high as you can. Land softly and go back into a squat.
- ☐ Bicycle Crunches: Lie on your back with your hands behind your head.

  Alternately, bring your opposite elbow to the opposite knee in a bicycle pedal motion.
- ☐ Plank Hold: Get into a forearm plank position and hold it for the designated time.

5. **Cool-Down:**

- ☐ Finish the workout with 5–10 minutes of light stretching, focusing on the muscles you worked during the HIIT session.

Remember to listen to your body, modify the exercises as needed, and stay hydrated throughout the workout. This HIIT routine helps increase blood flow, promote detoxification through sweating, reduce stress, and improve overall circulation, all of which can contribute to a healthy and glowing complexion.

Exercise 3: Resistance Training

Are you ready to take your fitness game to the next level? Incorporating resistance training exercises, like weightlifting or bodyweight exercises, into your routine will be a game-changer for building muscle and improving your body composition. And guess what? Your skin will thank you too!

Resistance training is like giving your muscles a wake-up call. When you challenge your muscles by lifting weights or engaging in bodyweight exercises, you're stimulating muscle growth and increasing muscle tone. This not only helps you achieve that sculpted, toned look but also has a positive impact on your skin.

Here's a routine you can try (feel free to start with fewer repetitions and increase them gradually).

☐ **Warm-Up**:

Start with 5–10 minutes of light cardio, such as jogging in place or jumping jacks, to warm-up your muscles and increase blood flow.

☐ **Squats:**

Stand with your feet shoulder-width apart, place the resistance band just above your knees, and secure it in place. Lower your body down into a squat position, keeping your chest lifted and knees tracking over your toes. Push through your heels to return to the starting position. Aim for three sets of 10–12 repetitions.

☐ **Push-Ups:**

Assume a high plank position with the resistance band looped around your upper back, just below your shoulder blades. Perform push-ups, focusing on engaging your core and keeping your body in a straight line. If needed, modify by performing push-ups from your knees. Aim for three sets of 8–10 repetitions.

☐ **Resistance Band Rows:**

Anchor the resistance band to a sturdy object at waist height. Stand facing the anchor point, holding the band handles in your hands. Step back to create tension in the band, and maintain a slight bend in your knees. Pull the handles towards your body, squeezing your shoulder blades together. Return to the starting position with control. Aim for three sets of 10–12 repetitions.

☐ **Lunges:**

Stand with your feet hip-width apart, loop the resistance band around your ankles, and secure it in place. Take a big step forward with your right foot, lowering your body down into a lunge position. Push back up to the starting position and repeat on the other side. Aim for three sets of 10–12 repetitions on each leg.

- ☐ **Glute Bridges:**

  Lie on your back with your knees bent and feet flat on the ground. Place the resistance band just above your knees. Press your hips up towards the ceiling, engaging your glutes and hamstrings. Lower your hips back down to the ground with control. Aim for three sets of 12–15 repetitions.

- ☐ **Plank with Band Abduction:**

  Assume a high plank position with the resistance band looped around your ankles. While maintaining a stable core, lift one leg out to the side, opening your hip against the resistance of the band. Return the leg to the starting position and repeat on the other side. Aim for three sets of 8–10 repetitions on each side.

- ☐ **Cool-Down:**

  Finish your workout with some light stretching for each major muscle group, holding each stretch for 15–30 seconds.

Exercise 4: Pilates

Pilates is all about strengthening your core, improving flexibility, and developing body awareness. Through controlled movements and specific breathing techniques, Pilates engages multiple muscle groups. By practising Pilates, you can improve your posture, enhance circulation, and achieve an overall body tone, which can positively impact the appearance of your skin.

How can Pilates help you?

- **Enhanced Circulation**

One of the significant benefits of Pilates is its ability to improve circulation throughout the body. The controlled movements and muscle engagement in Pilates encourage blood flow to all areas, including the skin. With improved circulation, the skin receives a greater supply of oxygen, essential nutrients and immune cells. This nourishment supports the skin's health and vitality, promoting a radiant complexion and aiding in the repair and rejuvenation of skin cells. The increased blood flow also aids in the removal of toxins and waste products from the skin, contributing to a clearer and more vibrant appearance.

- **Stress Reduction**

Pilates is not just a physical exercise; it is a mind–body practice that emphasizes mindfulness and body awareness. Through focused breathing techniques and intentional movements, Pilates helps activate the body's relaxation response, reducing stress levels and promoting a sense of calm. Chronic stress can have detrimental effects on the skin, leading to inflammation, breakouts and accelerated ageing. By engaging in Pilates, you can effectively manage stress, minimizing its negative impact on the skin. The release of tension and the promotion of relaxation through Pilates can help restore balance in the body, improving overall well-being and promoting a healthy complexion.

Are you ready to start your Pilates routine? Consider incorporating the following exercises into your practice:

- ☐ **The Hundred**

  Lie on your back with your knees bent, and lift your head and shoulders off the mat. Extend your legs to a 45-degree angle and pump your arms up and down while inhaling for five counts and exhaling for five counts. Repeat for ten breaths.

- ☐ **Pilates Roll-Up**

  Begin by lying on your back with your arms extended overhead. Slowly roll up, reaching for your toes, and then roll back down one vertebra at a time. Aim for six to eight repetitions.

- ☐ **Pilates Plank**

  Assume a plank position with your hands directly under your shoulders and your body forming a straight line. Hold this position for a challenging yet manageable amount of time, gradually increasing as you build strength.

Exercise 5: Yoga

Yoga combines physical poses, breathing exercises, and meditation to promote a sense of balance and well-being. Certain yoga poses, like downward dog or shoulder stand, encourage blood flow to your face, nourishing your skin. Moreover, yoga's stress-reducing effects can indirectly benefit your skin by minimizing stress-related skin issues.

How will yoga help with your skin issues?

- ☐ **Detoxification**

Yoga plays a powerful role in supporting the body's natural detoxification processes. Certain yoga poses, such as twists and forward folds, stimulate the internal organs and massage the digestive system. These movements enhance blood flow to the organs involved in detoxification, such as the liver and kidneys. By promoting circulation and movement, yoga helps to flush out toxins and waste products from the body. This reduction in toxic load can have a positive impact on the skin, leading to a clearer complexion and a healthier overall appearance.

- ☐ **Relaxation and Stress Reduction**

Yoga is renowned for its ability to induce relaxation and reduce stress levels. Through the combination of mindful movements, controlled breathing, and meditation, yoga activates the body's relaxation response, triggering the parasympathetic nervous system. This shift from a state of stress to relaxation has a profound impact on skin health. Chronic stress can lead to inflammation, breakouts, and premature ageing. By practising yoga, you can lower stress hormone levels, such as cortisol, which helps rebalance the body and alleviate stress-related skin issues. The deep relaxation experienced during yoga promotes a sense of calm, supporting healthy skin from within.

Here are a few yoga asanas (yoga poses) that can help promote skin health:

Sarvangasana (Shoulder Stand): This inverted pose increases blood flow to the face and promotes a healthy glow. It also stimulates the thyroid gland, which plays a crucial role in regulating skin health. Start by lying on your back, lifting your legs up towards the ceiling, and supporting your lower back with your hands. Hold the pose for a few breaths and gradually increase the duration as you become more comfortable.

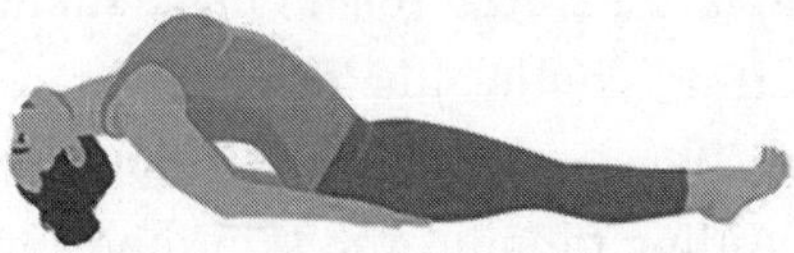

Matsyasana (Fish Pose): Matsyasana helps open up the chest, stretching the facial muscles and improving circulation to the face. Lie on your back, place your hands under your hips, and lift your chest by pressing down on your elbows. Tilt your head back and hold the pose while breathing deeply.

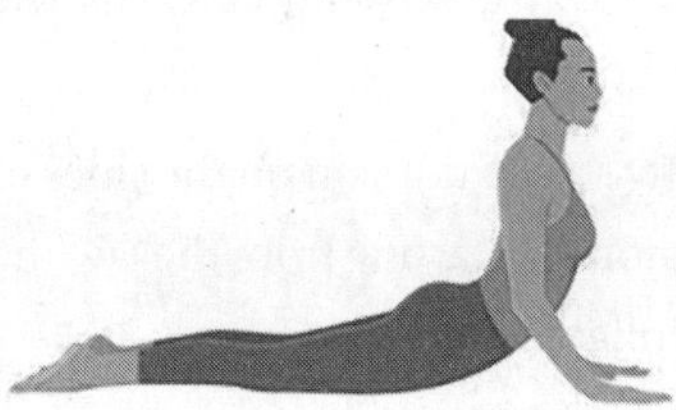

Uttanasana (Standing Forward Bend): Uttanasana helps increase blood flow to the face and promotes relaxation. Stand with your feet hip-width apart, fold forward from your hips, and let your head and neck relax. You can bend your knees if needed. Allow gravity to deepen the stretch and hold the pose for a few breaths.

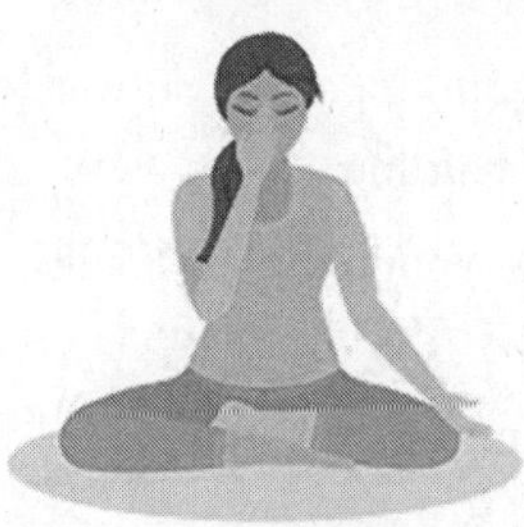

Pranayama (Breathing Exercises): Deep breathing exercises, such as kapalabhati (skull shining breath)

or anulom vilom (alternate nostril breathing), can help reduce stress, oxygenate the body, and promote healthy skin. Sit comfortably, close your eyes, and focus on your breath as you practise these techniques.

Lymphatic Drainage Exercise for Skin Health:

Lymphatic drainage exercises are designed to stimulate the lymphatic system, which plays a crucial role in maintaining overall health and supporting skin health. These exercises can help improve lymphatic flow, reduce fluid retention, and enhance detoxification, leading to improved skin tone and texture. Here's a simple lymphatic drainage exercise you can try:

Neck and Face Lymphatic Drainage:

1. Begin by sitting or standing in a comfortable position.
2. Gently tilt your head backward, looking towards the ceiling.
3. Using your fingertips, lightly stroke the skin on the sides of your neck in a downward motion, starting from the jawline and moving towards the collarbone.
4. Repeat this stroking motion 5–10 times.
5. Next, place your fingertips on your face, near the centre of your forehead.
6. Apply gentle pressure and move your fingertips outward in a circular motion, following the hairline.
7. Continue the circular motion across your temples, cheeks, and jawline.
8. Repeat this exercise for several minutes.

***If You Don't Have Time for Manual Lymphatic Drainage*:**

While manual lymphatic drainage exercises are beneficial, they can be time-consuming. If you find it challenging to incorporate these exercises into your routine, you can consider alternative therapies that involve complete lymphatic drainage, such as lymphatic drainage massage or lymphatic drainage machines. These therapies are performed by trained professionals and can help stimulate lymphatic flow, reduce fluid retention, and promote healthy skin. Consult with a qualified therapist or healthcare provider to explore these options further.

Remember, consistency is important for optimal results. Whether you choose to perform manual lymphatic drainage exercises or seek professional therapies, supporting your lymphatic system can contribute to healthier skin and overall well-being.

Vegetarian Diet Plan for Glowing Skin

Early morning: 1 glass of lukewarm water with 1 tsp of apple cider vinegar and 1 tsp of turmeric

Breakfast: 1 glass of green smoothie

Mid-morning: 1 seasonal fruit

Lunch: 1 bowl dal, 1 bowl seasonal vegetable, 1 ragi roti, 1 bowl curd, salad and pickle

Evening snack: 1 cup of herbal detox tea by Nutracy Lifestyle with 1 snack (a protein bar) by Nutracy Lifestyle

Dinner: Tomato cashewnut soup with makhana bhel

Non-vegetarian Diet Plan for Glowing Skin

Early morning: 1 glass of luke warm water with 1 tsp of A2 cow ghee

Breakfast:

Option 1: 1 glass of red smoothie

Option 2: 1 glass of green smoothie

Lunch:

Option 1: Tandoori chicken with brown rice and mixed salad

Option 2: Grilled salmon with quinoa and roasted vegetables

Snacks: 1 glass of beauty collagen drink

Dinner:

Option 1: Fish curry with quinoa and sautéed spinach

Option 2: 2 whole egg curries with stir-fried vegetables

GROCERY LIST

- ☐ Quinoa
- ☐ Bajra (whole, flour)
- ☐ Jowar (whole, flour)
- ☐ Red lentils (masoor dal)
- ☐ Bengal gram dal (chana dal)
- ☐ Black gram dal (urad dal)
- ☐ Chickpea (chole)
- ☐ Almond milk/ A2 cow's milk
- ☐ Plain curd/yoghurt
- ☐ Sunflower seeds
- ☐ Walnuts
- ☐ Flaxseeds
- ☐ Black cumin seeds
- ☐ Guava

- ☐ Kiwi
- ☐ Oranges
- ☐ Papaya
- ☐ Strawberries
- ☐ Watermelon with seeds
- ☐ Apple
- ☐ Muskmelon
- ☐ Pomegranate
- ☐ Carrots
- ☐ Beetroot
- ☐ Cucumber
- ☐ Tomato
- ☐ Pumpkin
- ☐ Spinach
- ☐ Lettuce
- ☐ Bell peppers
- ☐ Broccoli
- ☐ French beans
- ☐ Olive oil/coconut oil/ghee
- ☐ Salmon
- ☐ Eggs
- ☐ Chicken
- ☐ Collagen powder by Nutracy Lifestyle

The power of infrared lights on your skin

Light therapy, also known as phototherapy, is a non-invasive treatment method that utilizes specific wavelengths of light to address various skin concerns. It has gained popularity as a safe and effective approach for improving the overall health and appearance of the skin.

One common type of light therapy is LED (light-emitting diode) therapy. LED devices emit different colours of light, such as red, blue, and yellow, which penetrate the skin at varying depths to target specific skin issues. Here are some benefits and uses of light therapy for the skin:

1. **Acne Treatment:** Blue light therapy is often used to treat acne. It works by targeting and destroying acne-causing bacteria, reducing inflammation, and promoting a clearer complexion. Several studies have demonstrated the effectiveness of blue light therapy in reducing acne lesions. For instance, a study published in the *Journal of Clinical and Aesthetic Dermatology* found that blue light therapy significantly reduced acne lesions by up to 67 per cent after eight weeks of treatment.

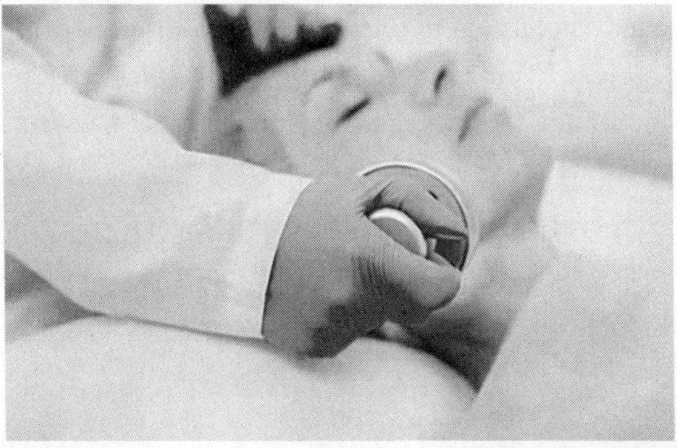

2. **Skin Rejuvenation:** Red light therapy is commonly used for skin rejuvenation and anti-ageing purposes. It stimulates collagen production, improves skin elasticity, and reduces the appearance of fine lines and wrinkles. Research published in the journal *Seminars in Cutaneous Medicine and Surgery* shows that red light therapy can improve skin texture, increase collagen density, and enhance overall skin tone.

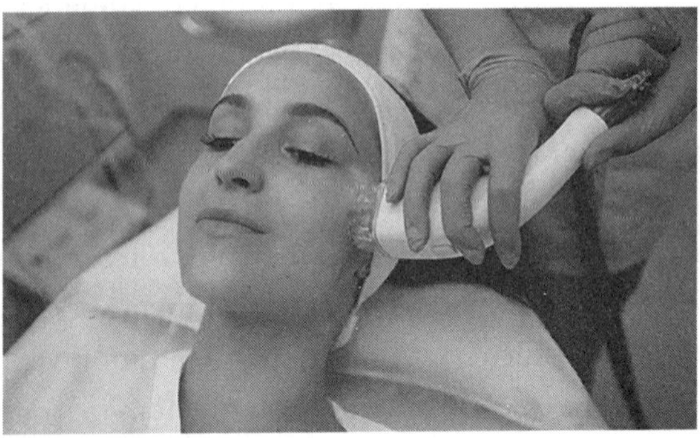

3. **Wound Healing:** Light therapy, particularly with red and near-infrared light, has shown promising results in promoting wound healing. These wavelengths of light penetrate deep into the skin and stimulate cellular processes that facilitate tissue repair and regeneration. A study published in the journal *Photomedicine and Laser Surgery* found that red light therapy accelerated wound healing and reduced inflammation in patients with chronic wounds.
4. **Hyperpigmentation and Scarring:** Light therapy can also help reduce hyperpigmentation, such as dark spots and

melasma, by targeting excess melanin production in the skin. Additionally, it can aid in minimizing the appearance of scars and improving skin tone. A study published in the *Journal of Cosmetic Dermatology* reported that a combination of red and yellow light therapy effectively reduced post-inflammatory hyperpigmentation and improved overall skin complexion.

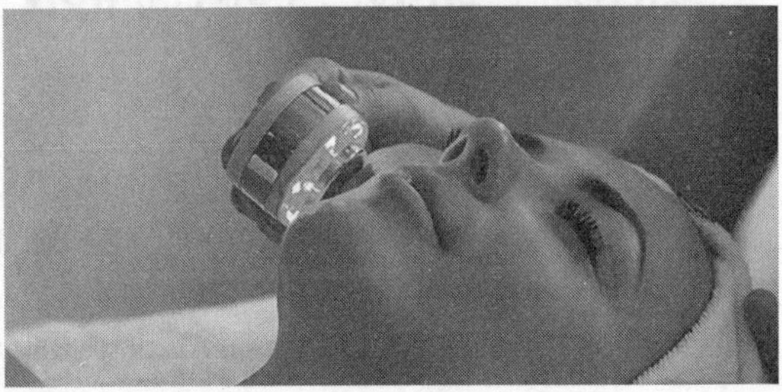

SKINCARE GUIDE: CONCLUSION

- In conclusion, skincare nutrition is a vital aspect of maintaining healthy, radiant, and youthful skin. A well-balanced diet rich in essential nutrients plays a significant role in supporting skin health and appearance.
- Key nutrients such as vitamins A, C, E and D, along with antioxidants like selenium and zinc, are essential for promoting collagen production, protecting the skin from oxidative damage, and maintaining its elasticity and suppleness. Omega-3 fatty acids help nourish the skin, reduce inflammation, and support skin barrier function.
- Including a variety of colourful fruits, vegetables, whole grains, nuts, seeds, and lean proteins in the diet can provide a wide range of these essential nutrients. Hydration is equally important for skin health, so drinking enough water throughout the day is essential.
- On the other hand, limiting the intake of processed foods, sugary beverages, and foods high in unhealthy fats

can help prevent skin issues such as acne and premature ageing.

- While nutrition is an important factor, it is equally essential to protect the skin from external factors like harmful UV rays, pollution, and excessive sun exposure. Adopting a consistent skincare routine and using appropriate sunscreen can help safeguard the skin from damage.
- Remember that everyone's skin is unique, and individual needs may vary. Consulting with dermatologists or registered dietitians can offer personalized advice, considering specific skin concerns and health conditions.
- By embracing a holistic approach to skincare nutrition, combining a balanced diet, proper hydration, and a suitable skincare routine, we can nurture our skin from the inside out, revealing a glowing, healthy complexion that reflects overall well-being.

BIBLIOGRAPHY

1. Baumann, L. (2009). Cosmetic Dermatology: Principles and Practice (2nd ed.). McGraw-Hill Medical.
2. Danby, F. W. (2010). Nutrition and acne. *Clinics in Dermatology,* 28(6), 598-604.
3. Katta, R., & Desai, S. P. (2014). Diet and dermatology: The role of dietary intervention in skin disease. *Journal of Clinical and Aesthetic Dermatology,* 7(7), 46-51.Schagen, S. K., Zampeli, V. A., Makrantonaki, E., & Zouboulis, C. C. (2012).
4. Discovering the link between nutrition and skin aging. *Dermato-Endocrinology,* 4(3), 298-307.
5. Veith, W. B., & Silverberg, N. B. (2011). The association of acne vulgaris with diet. Cutis, 88(2), 84-91.
6. Zhou J, Dong Y, Liu J, Ren J, Wu J, Zhu N. AQP5 regulates the proliferation and differentiation of epidermal stem cells in skin ageing. *Braz J Med Biol Res.* 2020 Sep 18;53(11):e10009. doi: 10.1590/1414-431X202010009. PMID: 32965322; PMCID: PMC7510230.

7. National Institutes of Health (NIH) Office of Dietary Supplements: Website providing comprehensive information on vitamins, minerals and dietary supplements. (ods.od.nih.gov)
8. Academy of Nutrition and Dietetics: Professional organisation for dietitians and nutritionists offering evidence-based information on nutrition and health. (www.eatright.org)
9. American Academy of Dermatology: Official website of the organisation providing resources on skin health, including nutrition's impact on skin. (www.aad.org)
10. World Health Organization (WHO): International health organisation with resources on nutrition and health. (www.who.int)
11. *The Journal of Investigative Dermatology*: Scientific journal publishing research on various aspects of dermatology, including skin nutrition. (www.jidonline.org)
12. *The Journal of the American Academy of Dermatology*: Peer-reviewed journal with articles on dermatology and skin-related research. (www.jaad.org)
13. Byrd, A., Belkaid, Y. & Segre, J. The human skin microbiome. Nat Rev Microbiol **16**, 143–155 (2018). https://doi.org/10.1038/nrmicro.2017.157
14. National Library of Medicine (PubMed): Online database with a vast collection of scientific articles on nutrition and skin/hair health. (pubmed.ncbi.nlm.nih.gov)

PART- 2

THE HAIRCARE GUIDE

INTRODUCTION

Hair is an integral part of our appearance, contributing to our overall confidence and sense of self. Achieving a great haircut, colour, and style can enhance our appearance and boost our confidence. However, caring for our hair is a complex matter that goes beyond simply using shampoo and conditioner. The foods we consume also play a significant role in maintaining hair health and ensuring its remarkable appearance.

A healthy diet is not only crucial for our overall well-being but also for the health of our hair. Certain nutrients are essential for strong, lustrous hair, and incorporating them into our daily diet can significantly improve its condition. In this book, we will explore two of the most important nutrients for healthy hair and provide guidance on how to include them in your diet effectively.

While using hair products can be beneficial, it's important to exercise caution, especially if you aspire to grow your hair long. Many hair products contain chemicals that, over time, can cause damage to your hair, particularly if you have thin or fine hair.

Furthermore, excessive use of products can lead to build-up and make your hair appear oily, which is especially problematic for those with oily skin.

Proper haircare is an essential part of maintaining overall health. Just like any other organ in our body, our hair requires proper care and nourishment to stay healthy. Neglecting the nutritional aspect of haircare can contribute to frequent damage. The foods we consume can either nurture or harm our hair, making it crucial to pay attention to our dietary habits.

It's not sufficient to rely solely on hairstyling techniques and products. To ensure optimal hair health, we must also prioritize proper nutrition. In the following sections, we will delve deeper into the significance of hair nutrition and explore the specific nutrients that promote healthy hair growth and prevent damage. By understanding the role of nutrition in haircare, you'll be equipped with the knowledge to make informed choices and embrace a holistic approach to maintaining vibrant, luscious hair.

Chapter 1

WHAT DOES NUTRITION HAVE TO DO WITH HAIR?

As you would know, what you eat has a direct impact on the health and appearance of your lovely locks. It's like a delicious recipe where the right ingredients create a masterpiece in your head. So, let's dive into the magical connection between nutrition and hair health, with a sprinkle of Indian traditional wisdom and a dash of grandma's love.

In Indian culture, hair is often referred to as 'crowning glory'. Our ancestors believed that our hair is not just a mere fashion statement but a reflection of our overall well-being. They understood that true beauty starts from within, and that includes nourishing our bodies with the right foods. Our grandmas would lovingly oil our hair, not just for its shine but as a symbol of care and attention to our health.

When it comes to nutrition and hair, the numbers speak for themselves. Did you know that our hair is made up of a protein called keratin? It's like the building blocks of a strong and resilient fortress. So, it's no wonder that protein-rich foods like lean meats, eggs, dairy products and pulses are crucial for healthy hair growth. They provide the essential amino acids needed to maintain those luscious locks.

How Will Your Food Affect Your Hair?

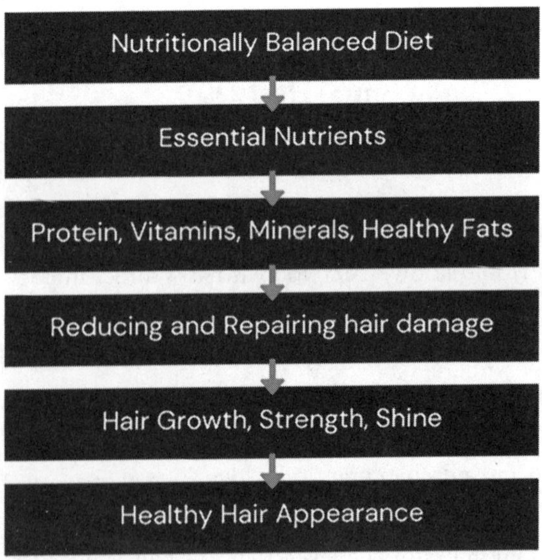

Growth and hair quality are maintained by a regular diet of amino acids, vitamins and minerals. The hair is composed of three main parts: scalp, hair shaft and root (hair bulb). The scalp is the part where your hair starts, and the base of the hair is where it attaches to your skull.

Taking proper care of your scalp will promote healthy hair growth.

To take the best care of your hair, it's important to start at the root and work your way up. Think of your hair roots as the foundation for healthy hair. They store all the essential nutrients needed for growth and vitality. By focusing on root care, you can nourish your hair from the inside out and prevent damage.

STRUCTURE OF THE HAIR

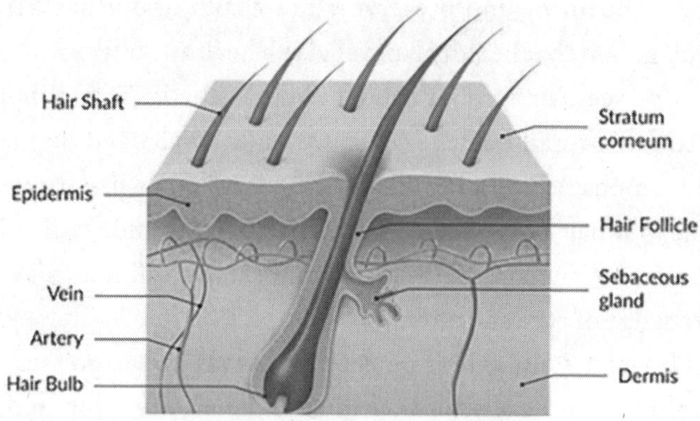

The main function of hair is to protect the scalp from the sun and wind as well as keep the skin moisturized. So, we need to take good care of our hair from a nutrition point of view too. Nutrition plays an important role when it comes to haircare because it can affect how much shine your hair has and whether or not it looks healthy overall.

The secret to healthy hair lies in **what you eat and drink.** Your daily diet must include all the necessary elements for healthy growth and function: proteins, vitamins, minerals and omega-3 fatty acids (for example, spinach). A balanced diet will not only help prevent hair loss but also make it grow faster, stronger and healthier!

In Indian households, grandmas have always been the guardians of haircare secrets. They would lovingly prepare concoctions with ingredients like hibiscus, amla (Indian gooseberry) and coconut oil, creating potions that would transform our hair into cascading waves of beauty. These age-old rituals were not just about superficial beauty but about nurturing and preserving the health of our hair. They understood that healthy hair reflects a healthy body.

You see, hair is not just about visual aesthetics; it's a window into our overall health. When we have a balanced diet rich in vitamins A, C, D and E, along with minerals like iron and zinc, our hair rewards us with strength, shine, and vitality. It's like a love language between our bodies and our hair, a sweet exchange of care and attention.

Imagine your hair as a beautiful canvas that expresses the health of your body. Just as an artist needs the right colours and brushes to create a masterpiece, your body needs the right nutrients to paint a picture of vibrant and healthy hair. So, let's embark on this journey together, exploring the wonders of nutrition and its transformative effects on your precious tresses.

Remember, nourishing your hair is an act of self-love. It's a way of showing gratitude to your body, which works tirelessly to keep you strong and healthy. So, grab a cup of tea, sit back, and let's uncover the secrets of hair nutrition that will leave you feeling not just fabulous but radiantly healthy from head to toe.

Remember

A proper diet plays a crucial role in maintaining healthy hair since it affects every aspect of its growth process, from its initial creation to its destruction via styling products or cuts from grooming tools. A balanced diet promotes optimal blood flow for new growth which keeps hair shiny and strong. Such healthy hair will not produce knots or tangles which occur due to excess protein or insufficient essential vitamins. Unhealthy hair is difficult to style; bald spots or other unwanted effects on the scalp that would also cause premature hair destruction.

CHAPTER 2

HOW DOES AGEING AFFECT HAIR?

Normal hair growth involves the formation of new cells in the hair bulb, which is the root of the hair follicle. These new cells mature into functional units called hairs, which then grow out to form a healthy and strong scalp.

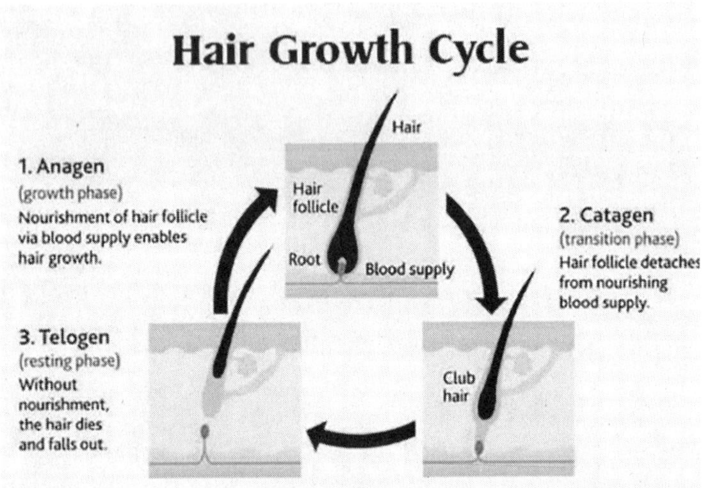

The Cycle of Normal Hair Growth

1. **Anagen phase:** Growth phase: The anagen phase lasts two to three years, during which time you have a lot of growing to do. Your hair grows approximately half an inch per month during this phase.
2. **Catagen phase**: Transition zone: This is the shortest phase (4 weeks) in which the hair shaft detaches from its roots to move into a resting stage called telogen. At this time, your scalp starts regenerating, so no more shedding!
3. **Telogen phase**: Resting phase: During telogen, cells from your body are used to replace those shed during catagen; these will soon be replaced by new hairs as they grow out from their follicles every twenty-eight days during telogen!

Changes in Hair Due to Ageing

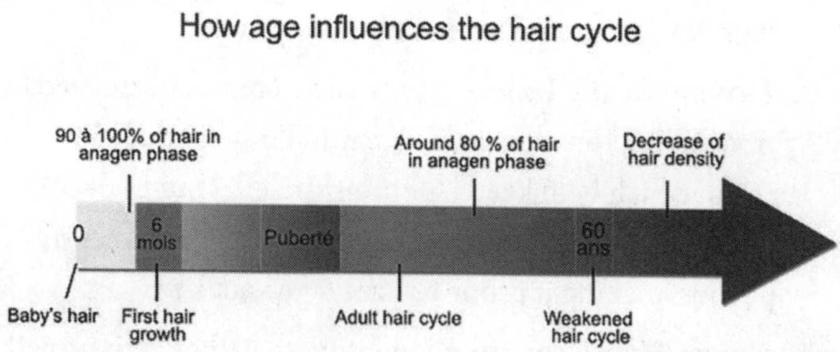

Hair growth is a fascinating process that goes through distinct phases known as the hair growth cycle. Understanding these phases can provide valuable insights into the dynamics of hair growth and the changes that occur in our hair over time. From luscious locks to the inevitable signs of ageing, our hair reflects the intricate balance between genetics, hormones, and environmental factors.

By delving into the intricacies of the hair growth phases, we can gain a deeper understanding of how these phases relate to the changes we observe in our hair as we age.

1. **Grey Hair:** One of the most visible signs of ageing hair is the development of grey hair. As we age, the cells responsible for producing pigment in our hair follicles begin to decline. This leads to a decrease in melanin production, resulting in hair strands that appear grey or white.
2. **Thinning Hair**: Another common effect of ageing on hair is thinning. As we get older, the rate of hair growth slows down, and hair follicles may become smaller and produce finer hair strands. This can lead to a noticeable decrease in hair density and volume.
3. **Dry and Brittle Hair**: Ageing hair is often characterized by dryness and brittleness. The natural oils produced by the scalp, which help keep hair moisturized, tend to decrease with age. Additionally, the hair shaft itself becomes more porous, making it prone to breakage and frizz.
4. **Slower Hair Growth**: As mentioned earlier, hair growth slows down with age. The growth phase of hair, known as the anagen phase, becomes shorter, leading to slower hair growth overall. This can contribute to thinning hair and a decrease in hair length.

5. **Texture Changes**: Many people also experience changes in hair texture as they age. Straight hair may become wavier or curlier, while curly hair may become less defined. These changes are believed to be due to alterations in the hair follicle structure.

Hair Thinning Due to Hormonal Changes

Hair is the most common body part to suffer from thinning. It is estimated that one out of every three people has a bald spot on the crown of their head. Baldness is caused by a number of factors, including heredity, age, hormones, stress and even certain types of medication.

There are many causes of hair loss, but not everyone suffers from the same type of condition. Some people lose their hair due to genetic conditions or other medical problems, such as alopecia areata or anaemia. Other people may experience hair loss as a result of poor nutrition or hygiene.

Oxidative Stress and Grey Hair

As you have read above, grey hair is one of the signs of ageing. As we age, our hair colour becomes duller and our skin loses its youthful glow. This happens because of a natural process called melanin production. Melanin is a substance that gives skin its colour and protects it from sunlight. The more you expose yourself to the sun, the more melanin your skin will produce.

But hey! Don't keep blaming sun exposure for damaging your hair and skin!

Everything needs balance—not just your diet but your lifestyle habits too. Not to mention, the sun is your source of

90 per cent of your daily vitamin D. It would be damaging to you only if you were regularly in the sun and not taking care of your hydration.

Oxidative damage is caused by free radicals, which are atoms or molecules with an unpaired electron. Free radicals can cause damage to DNA and proteins in cells, and these damaged cells may become cancerous. Grey hair can be caused by oxidative damage, which causes the hair to appear grey.

When there are too many free radicals in your body, they attack your melanin-producing cells and wear them down faster than they normally would. This process creates natural-looking greys in your hair that may seem like they have always been there!

But don't worry. Having grey hair does not mean you are prematurely ageing. Just keep an eye on the possible reasons for oxidative stress in your body. Grey hair is not necessarily a sign of premature ageing; it's just a product of the way your body reacts to stress and environmental factors. It can be caused by exposure to sunlight, smoking, pollution and other sources of oxidative stress.

Summary

Ageing affects hair in several ways. Grey hair occurs as melanin production declines, while hair thinning and reduced density are common due to slower growth and shrinking hair follicles. Hair may become drier and more brittle, and changes in texture can occur. Additionally, oxidative stress plays a role in hair greying. Understanding these age-related changes can help individuals adapt their haircare routines and address specific concerns associated with ageing hair.

CHAPTER 3

GUT HEALTH AND HAIR CONNECTION

Gut health plays a crucial role in maintaining healthy hair, and it can be affected by both dietary issues and the immune system. Our hair relies on a balanced intake of macro and micronutrients from the diet to support its growth and maintain a normal hair cycle. However, for these nutrients to be effectively absorbed, they need to be broken down in the gut. If there's an imbalance in the digestive system, it can hinder nutrient absorption.

The connection between gut health and hair goes beyond just nutrition. A healthy gut is closely intertwined with a strong immune system and the proper balance of hormones in the body. When your hormones are functioning optimally, it promotes hair growth. Your gut bacteria also have a role to play in regulating hormone levels throughout your body, including those responsible for controlling the different phases of the hair growth cycle. Moreover, they can influence physical factors that affect blood flow to the skin and scalp. By maintaining a diet that supports gut health and creating an environment rich in beneficial bacteria, you can help create the optimal conditions for hair growth.

Inflammation in the Hair

Have you ever noticed small red bumps or white-headed pimples around hair follicles—the tiny pockets from which each hair grows? It is possibly due to inflammation in your body.

Nutrition plays a crucial role in maintaining healthy hair, and one of the key connections between nutrition and hair health lies in the condition of your gut. The health of your gut can have a significant impact on the appearance and vitality of your hair. It affects the absorption of essential nutrients and can influence the presence of inflammation in your body, which in turn affects your hair follicles.

When your gut is compromised or imbalanced, it can hinder the absorption of important nutrients necessary for healthy hair growth. Nutrients such as vitamins, minerals, and proteins need to be properly broken down and absorbed in the gut to support hair follicle function. If your digestive system is out of balance, it can disrupt this process, leading to nutrient deficiencies that can weaken your hair and impede its growth.

Furthermore, gut health is closely tied to inflammation throughout your body, including the scalp. Chronic inflammation can disrupt the normal hair growth cycle and contribute to hair loss, thinning, and scalp conditions. An imbalanced gut microbiota can promote inflammation, triggering an immune response that negatively affects hair follicles. This can result in conditions like scalp psoriasis, seborrhoeic dermatitis or folliculitis, which can cause hair-related problems.

Not just the gut, but our hair follicles have their own group of healthy bacteria too.

These are the most abundant bacteria present in your scalp and can be affected by your inflammatory diet.

Bacteria	How Does It Affect Us?	What Can You Do?
Burkholderia	Can affect immuno compromised people and cause infections on the scalp [PMID: 32295766]	Drink purified water and maintain hygiene
Staphylococcus	Can produce scarring alopecia (folliculitis decalvans) in middle-aged adults [PMID: 19295051]	Improve nutritional intake, especially vitamin A and B3
Cutibacterium	Increases sebum production and leads to dandruff [PMID: 33790324]	Correct biotin levels Apply coconut oil to the scalp

Inflammation of the Gut and Hair Damage

When it comes to our overall health, the gut plays a vital role, serving as a central hub for digestion, the absorption of nutrients, and even immune function. However, many are

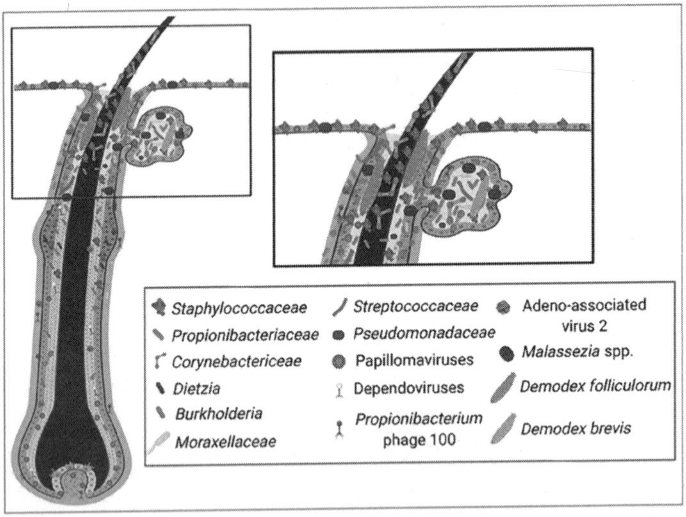

Bacteria seen in and around the hair follicles

unaware of the significant impact gut inflammation can have on our hair health.

The gut is an important part of the body's immune system. When it's inflamed, it can cause many different health conditions, including autoimmune diseases like lupus, Hashimoto's disease and multiple sclerosis. In these cases, the gut produces antibodies that attack the body's own tissues and organs, which can result in hair loss or thinning.

In addition to inflammation in the gut, there are also other factors that can cause **hair loss or thinning**. These include the following:

1. **Nutritional Deficiencies**

Protein:

Protein deficiency is a significant factor that can contribute to various hair issues. Our hair is predominantly composed of a protein called keratin, which provides strength, structure, and resilience to our strands. Thus, a deficiency in dietary protein can directly impact the health and appearance of our hair.

When our body lacks sufficient protein intake, it prioritizes vital functions over non-essential ones like hair growth. As a result, the hair follicles enter a resting phase known as the telogen phase, which causes hair shedding. This can lead to noticeable hair thinning, weakened strands, and an overall decrease in hair density.

Iron:

Iron deficiency can have a significant impact on hair health. Iron is a vital mineral that plays a crucial role in various bodily functions, including the growth and maintenance of hair follicles. When our body lacks sufficient iron, it can lead to a condition called iron deficiency anaemia, which can negatively affect the health and appearance of our hair.

One common hair-related symptom of iron deficiency is excessive hair shedding, known as telogen effluvium. This occurs when a large number of hair follicles enter the resting phase (telogen phase) prematurely and shed more than usual. As a result, individuals may notice increased hair thinning and a decrease in hair volume.

Furthermore, iron deficiency can affect the structure and quality of the hair. Without sufficient iron, hair strands may become brittle, dry, and prone to breakage. The hair may lose its shine and appear dull and lack lustre.

Omega-3 Fatty Acids:

Omega-3 deficiency can significantly impact hair health. These essential fatty acids play a crucial role in nourishing the hair follicles and maintaining a healthy scalp. When there is a lack of omega-3s in the diet, it can lead to various hair issues. One common problem is dry and brittle hair, as omega-3s help retain moisture in the hair strands, keeping them hydrated and resilient. Without sufficient omega-3s, the hair can become dry, dull, and prone to breakage.

Another consequence of omega-3 deficiency is increased hair shedding. Omega-3s possess anti-inflammatory properties that help reduce scalp inflammation. Inflammation in the scalp can disrupt the hair growth cycle, leading to excessive hair shedding and thinning. Additionally, omega-3s contribute to the strength and integrity of the hair follicles, making them less susceptible to damage. When there is a deficiency, the hair follicles may weaken, resulting in increased hair loss.

Biotin:

Biotin, also known as vitamin B7, is a critical nutrient for hair growth and strength. Inadequate biotin levels can lead to hair becoming brittle, experiencing increased hair loss, and even developing dermatitis.

Biotin deficiency can have significant implications for hair health. Biotin, also known as vitamin B7, is essential for the production of keratin, the protein that forms the structure of hair strands. When the body lacks sufficient biotin, it can result in hair thinning, increased hair loss, and slow hair growth. Additionally, biotin plays a role in maintaining the moisture balance of the hair, and a deficiency can lead to dry, brittle hair that is more prone to breakage. Furthermore, inadequate biotin levels may contribute to scalp issues such as dryness, flakiness, and itching, which can further compromise the overall health and appearance of the hair.

However, it is important to note that biotin deficiency is relatively rare among individuals who maintain a well-balanced diet.

Zinc:

Zinc deficiency can have detrimental effects on hair health, leading to various hair problems. Zinc is an essential mineral that plays a vital role in cell division and protein synthesis, which are essential processes for hair growth. When the body lacks adequate zinc levels, it can disrupt the normal hair growth cycle, resulting in increased hair shedding and slower hair regrowth. Zinc deficiency has been linked to conditions such as telogen effluvium, where the hair prematurely enters the resting phase, leading to excessive hair loss.

Furthermore, zinc is involved in maintaining the health of the hair follicles and sebaceous glands. Insufficient zinc levels can disrupt the production of sebum, the natural oil that moisturizes the scalp and hair. This can lead to a dry scalp, dandruff and brittle hair that is prone to breakage. Additionally, zinc plays a role in immune function, and a weakened immune system due to zinc deficiency can contribute to scalp infections, further exacerbating hair problems.

In Chapter 7, we will delve into a deeper understanding of these remarkable nutrients. We will explore their intricate roles in supporting our overall health and well-being. From macronutrients like carbohydrates, proteins, and fats that provide us with energy, to micronutrients such as vitamins and minerals that aid in vital bodily functions, we will uncover the fascinating world of nutrition.

2. **Hormones**

Testosterone:

Hormonal imbalances, such as low testosterone levels, can lead to a number of hair issues and they can cause coordinating health issues as well. Age is another one of those common causes that you simply cannot do anything about. The older you are, the more likely you are to experience thinning hair or hair loss.

Hair loss is one of the most common complaints among men. It affects millions of men around the world and has a significant impact on their self-esteem.

The causes of hair loss are many and varied, but testosterone levels play a role in the condition. Testosterone is a male hormone that provides sexual characteristics, including hair growth. If your levels are low, you may have less than normal amounts of this hormone circulating in your body.

Cortisol:

One day you wake up from a nap to find your phone is not beside you, and you get anxious. You start looking for it everywhere, and your blood pressure increases. Why? The answer is cortisol.

It is the human stress hormone. Although cortisol can fluctuate on a daily basis, it will only count as a hormonal imbalance when it's constantly high throughout the day. When it is present at high levels, it reduces the production and regeneration of an important element called hyaluronan and proteoglycans by approximately forty per cent. These elements are very essential for healthy hair and to prevent hair damage.

Follicle Stimulating Hormone (FSH):

The follicle-stimulating hormone (FSH) is responsible for stimulating hair growth. When an overactive FSH occurs, it can cause thinning of one's hair and even hair loss. One of the most common causes of a hormonal imbalance that can lead to hair loss is stress.

Men and women who have low levels of FSH will experience hair loss as they age. Some people call it male-pattern baldness or female-pattern baldness.

Stress can affect hormones like FSH in a number of ways. It can lead to an increase in cortisol levels, which makes it harder for testosterone to function properly, thus leading to less production of DHT, or dihydrotestosterone, by the body, which is responsible for causing hair loss and baldness.

Melatonin:

Melatonin is a hormone that is produced in the pineal gland and secreted into the brain. Melatonin levels increase at night and decrease during the day. This change in melatonin levels is one of many factors that control sleep rhythms.

It is an indirect helper hormone in preventing hair loss. See, we all know that as we age, our sleep is disturbed largely. Look at our parents and grandparents; they are always ready to wake up early and sleep late! Well, now you know that it's a sign that their melatonin levels have been affected.

Also, did anyone else notice that our mothers and grandmothers often have short hair or a sleek braid with very thinned-down hair?

Well, melatonin is to blame here too!

Research says that the hormone is both directly and indirectly related to hair growth.

Recent medical research from Harvard Medical School and the American Academy of Dermatology [6] indicates that chronic inflammation can lead to symptoms such as the following:

- Shrinking of the hair follicle
- Reduced hair volume
- Thinning hair

Hair loss and hair damage—both are not something we want, right?

But the reality is that the inflammation in your body can harm your hair and cause both of the above.

Stress and Inflammation

Stress triggers the release of cortisol, which can adversely affect hair follicles. Elevated cortisol levels can lead to hair thinning and, in severe cases, result in temporary hair loss (telogen effluvium). Managing stress and cortisol levels is essential for maintaining healthy hair.

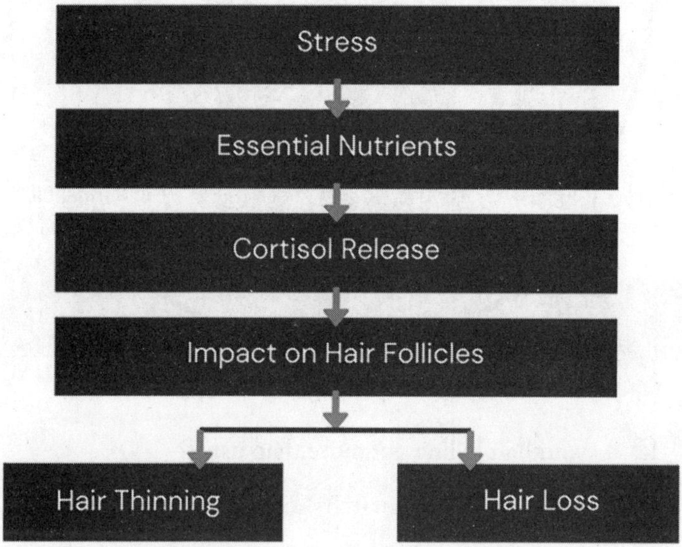

Relationship between Hair Loss and Gut Health

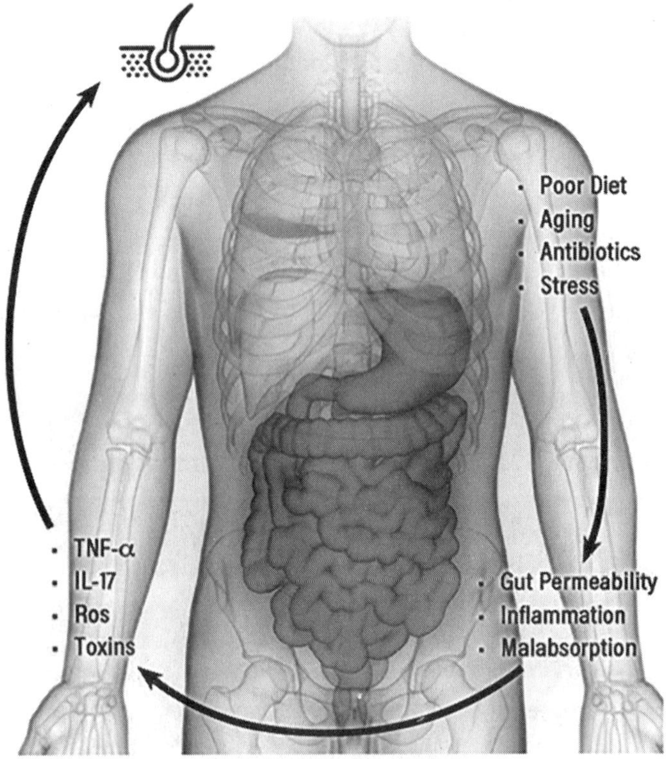

- ☐ Is your hair falling out more than usual?
- ☐ Do you experience an itchy scalp frequently?
- ☐ Are you troubled by excessive dandruff or flaking?
- ☐ Do you notice any redness, irritation or inflammation on your scalp?

- ☐ Have you observed thinning or sparse areas on your scalp?
- ☐ Do you frequently experience dryness or oiliness on your scalp?
- ☐ Have you noticed any changes in the texture or appearance of your hair?
- ☐ Do you have any scalp conditions, such as psoriasis or eczema?
- ☐ Are you experiencing any discomfort or pain on your scalp?
- ☐ Have you recently undergone any hair treatments or procedures that may have affected the health of your hair and scalp?

Did you know that the health of your gut could be closely linked to the problem of hairfall?

If you ticked more than one of the above, it is time to talk about your gut health!

The gut–hair connection is very important because it has been found that if your gut bacteria are healthy, then your body will be healthy. And if your body is healthy, so is your hair.

You see, our gut is home to trillions of bacteria, collectively known as the gut microbiota. These microscopic superheroes play a vital role in keeping our bodies functioning at their best. When our gut bacteria are thriving and in harmony, our immune system becomes stronger, our digestion improves, and our overall well-being is enhanced.

Guess what?

All of these factors contribute to the health and vitality of our hair.

Recent research has unveiled an intriguing relationship between the two, highlighting the significant impact of our gut microbiota—the trillions of bacteria residing in our digestive system—on the health and appearance of our hair. Understanding this connection can provide valuable insights into how to tackle hairfall and promote healthier, more resilient hair.

By digging into these insights, we can get a clearer picture of how our gut health affects hairfall and find some practical strategies to tackle this common issue. So, let's dive in and explore the fascinating connection between gut health and hairfall!

Several studies have explored this connection and uncovered some important findings that we can easily understand:

1. **Gut Microbiota and Hair Disorders**

Scientists have discovered that having a well-balanced gut microbiota is crucial for maintaining healthy hair. When the bacteria in our gut are in harmony, it can positively influence our hair health. Some studies have even suggested that taking probiotics or prebiotics, which help promote a healthy gut, may improve the condition of our hair.

2. **Gut Dysbiosis and Hair Growth**

Gut dysbiosis, which refers to an imbalance in the gut bacteria, has been associated with disrupted hair growth cycles and increased hairfall. Conditions like dandruff, alopecia areata, and thinning hair have been linked to an unhealthy gut microbiota. By restoring a healthy balance of gut bacteria through specific interventions, such as taking probiotics or adjusting our diet, we may be able to support hair growth and reduce hairfall.

3. **Gut Health and Nutrient Absorption**

A healthy gut microbiota plays a crucial role in absorbing and metabolizing nutrients, which are essential for maintaining healthy hair. When our gut is functioning well, it ensures that we absorb all the necessary nutrients that support hair growth. On the other hand, an imbalanced gut can hinder nutrient absorption, potentially leading to hairloss and compromised hair health.

Five Reasons Why Healing Your Gut Might Be Difficult for You

After delving into the intriguing relationship between hairfall and gut health, it becomes evident that nurturing a healthy gut is not always a simple task. The healing process can be influenced by several factors that pose challenges along the way, ultimately impacting the health and resilience of our hair. It is important to recognize and address these factors to maximize the effectiveness of gut healing efforts and promote improved hair health.

1. **You are only looking at digestive problems:** Digestive problems are not the only symptoms of a bad gut. Many people with digestive issues also have joint pain, brain fog, headaches and fatigue, among other symptoms. Here are a few more ways that you can identify if you have gut issues:
    - Intolerance or indigestion after certain foods
    - Recently noticeable allergies
    - Constantly feeling like resting most of the days
    - Feeling thirsty always but drinking water only when you feel extreme thirst
    - You sleep enough but still do not feel fresh when you wake up.

If you suspect that your gut health is suffering due to a poor diet, it's time to get to the root of the problem and start eating healthier.

2. **You are not aware of the deficiencies you might have:** Nutrient deficiencies and hair problems are among the most common complaints. The first thing is to determine if there is a nutrient deficiency, hormonal imbalance or other organic condition that is causing the problem. If this is not the case, we will proceed to treat the underlying cause.
    - **Vitamins A, C and E:** Vitamins A, C and E are antioxidants that help protect hair against free radical damage caused by pollution, UV rays or other environmental factors. These vitamins also help prevent

dryness, flaking and shedding of hair when applied topically.

- **B-complex vitamins:** Hair is made up of four layers. The top layer, the cuticle, is dead and in the process of transforming into the next generation. The middle layer, the cortex, contains pigment and keratin protein that makes hair strong and resilient. The bottom layer, the medulla or sheath, is where blood vessels are located and where blood can be stored for later use to nourish the cortex.

  For your hair to grow healthy and strong, it needs all three layers of your scalp to be in good health. The B-complex vitamins are essential for keeping this balance going.

3. **Your diet is not rich in fibre:** The fibre in your diet can help prevent hairfall and hair thinning. Fibre contains minerals like iron, zinc and manganese, which are essential for healthy hair. Fibre also helps in the growth of hair follicles and stimulates new cell production.

   The amount of fibre in your diet can make a difference to how well your hair looks after you've shed its protective outer layer (the cuticle). It's thought that people with low levels of dietary fibre tend to lose more hair during their lifetime than those with high levels.

   You will read more in detail about what nutrients you might be lacking in your daily diet for healthy hair in Chapter 7.

Case Study: 1

Client Profile	
Age	32 years
Gender	Female

Medical Complications	
Existing conditions	Vitamin D deficiency
Hair-related concern	Significant hair loss

Other Complaints	
Scalp symptoms	Itchy scalp and excessive dandruff
Hair condition	Thinning and sparse areas on the scalp

Existing Diet and Exercise	
Diet	Mainly processed foods and lack of fresh fruits and vegetables
Exercise	A sedentary lifestyle and lack of regular exercise

Recommendations and Interventions	
Dietary changes	Emphasized nutrient-rich foods such as fruits, vegetables, lean proteins, and whole grains, with a focus on foods high in

	calcium along with appropriate dosage of vitamin D supplements.
Gut health improvement	Incorporate probiotic-rich foods and consider a probiotic supplement
Lifestyle modifications	Encourage regular physical activity and exercise
Professional support	Consultation with a nutritionist and dermatologist

Improvement in Hair	
Hair loss reduction	After three months of following the recommended dietary and lifestyle changes, she observed a significant reduction in hair loss.
Scalp health improvement	The itchy scalp, excessive dandruff, and thinning areas showed improvement.
Hair regrowth	She noticed new hair growth in previously sparse areas.
Overall well-being	Alongside the improvement in hair, she reported feeling more energized and healthier.

Summary

In this chapter, we explored the intriguing connection between gut-health and hair. A healthy gut, supported by a balanced gut microbiota and proper nutrient absorption, is crucial for maintaining healthy hair. We discovered that imbalances in the gut, inflammation, nutritional deficiencies, and hormonal fluctuations can all contribute to hair problems such as hair loss, thinning, scalp inflammation, and dandruff. By understanding and addressing these factors through dietary changes, gut health improvement, and lifestyle modifications, we can promote healthier hair and overall well-being.

CHAPTER 4

IMPORTANCE OF MENTAL HEALTH FOR HEALTHY HAIR

Treating symptoms of anxiety and depression as soon as they begin can help you prevent mental health problems that lead to more hair loss.

In today's challenging times, many individuals are still grappling with significant financial and psychological burdens brought about by the ongoing pandemic. Amidst this turmoil, an unfortunate and intricate relationship exists between psychological distress and hair loss, forming a vicious cycle that further compounds the difficulties faced by individuals.

Hair loss, a widespread issue, can stem from a variety of factors, making it challenging to pinpoint a singular cause. However, in this chapter, we will delve into the connection between mental health and hair loss, exploring whether there is a link between the two.

While there are various primary causes of hair loss, it is essential to recognize that certain aspects of our lives can impact the health of our hair. Factors such as our diet, geographical location, alcohol consumption, stress levels and even our sleep patterns can all play a role in contributing to hair loss.

- ***Diet***, for instance, plays a crucial role in nurturing our bodies and, consequently, our hair. The nutrients we consume, or lack thereof, can influence the strength, vitality, and overall health of our hair follicles. Similarly, environmental factors, such as living in areas with high pollution levels or extreme climates, can affect the condition of our hair, making it more susceptible to damage and loss.
- ***Alcohol consumption***, particularly excessive or chronic intake, can also impact hair health. Alcohol can disrupt the normal functioning of the hair growth cycle and lead to increased hair shedding. Additionally, it can contribute to dehydration, which can negatively affect the moisture balance of the scalp and hair.
- ***Stress***, a common factor in modern-day life, can have a profound impact on hair loss. When our bodies experience prolonged or severe stress, it can disrupt the natural hair growth cycle. This disruption may cause hair follicles to prematurely enter the resting phase, leading to increased hair shedding and thinning. Moreover, stress-induced hormonal imbalances can further exacerbate the problem, creating a detrimental cycle for hair health.

- ***Sleep***, often overlooked but crucial for our overall well-being, also plays a role in maintaining healthy hair. Inadequate sleep or irregular sleep patterns can disrupt the body's natural regenerative processes, including hair growth. A lack of quality sleep can lead to increased stress levels and hormonal imbalances, both of which can contribute to hair loss.

  Exploring the impact of mental health on hair loss, we find a complex relationship between the two. Psychological distress, such as anxiety and depression, can manifest in physical symptoms, including **changes in hair quality and quantity**. Chronic anxiety, for example, can lead to a condition called trichotillomania, where individuals unconsciously pull out their hair as a coping mechanism, resulting in noticeable hair loss.

Understanding and addressing the mental health aspect of hair loss is crucial for holistic well-being. Seeking support from mental health professionals, practising stress-management techniques, and engaging in self-care activities can help alleviate the emotional burdens that may contribute to hair loss. By taking care of our mental health, we can create a positive environment for our hair to thrive.

It is important to remember that our hair is not solely an aesthetic attribute but also a reflection of our overall health. By considering the impact of mental health on hair loss and adopting a comprehensive approach that includes both psychological and haircare, we can nurture healthy hair and enhance our overall well-being.

Impact of COVID-19 on Hair

The impact of COVID-19 infection on hair health has been a subject of interest and concern for individuals who have experienced the virus. While COVID-19 primarily affects the respiratory system, some people have reported experiencing changes in their hair following infection. Several factors may contribute to these hair-related issues in individuals recovering from COVID-19:

- **Telogen Effluvium of Illness**

  Telogen effluvium is a type of temporary hair shedding that occurs after a significant physical or emotional stressor, such as a severe illness or infection. COVID-19 infection can be a substantial stressor on the body, leading to disruptions in the hair growth cycle. This disruption can cause hair follicles to prematurely enter the telogen (resting) phase, leading to increased shedding of hair a few months after recovery. While this hair shedding can be distressing, it is usually temporary, and hair growth should resume as the body recovers.

- **Fever and Dehydration**

  During the course of a COVID-19 infection, individuals may experience fever and dehydration. Elevated body temperature and dehydration can impact hair health. Dehydration can lead to dryness and brittle hair, making it more prone to breakage. Proper hydration and care for the hair can help mitigate the effects of dehydration on hair health.

- **Medications**

  Some individuals with COVID-19 may receive medications during their treatment, such as antiviral drugs or steroids. Certain medications can have side effects that impact hair health. For example, some medications may cause hair thinning or loss as a side effect. It is essential for individuals to be aware of the potential side effects of medications and discuss any concerns with their health care provider.

- **Stress and Anxiety**

  Dealing with a COVID-19 infection and the associated uncertainties can be emotionally challenging and stressful. As mentioned earlier, stress can contribute to hair loss through telogen effluvium. Emotional stress and anxiety can also lead to habits like trichotillomania, where individuals unconsciously pull out their hair as a coping mechanism. This can result in noticeable hair loss in the affected areas.

- **Nutritional Deficiencies**

  During illness and recovery, individuals may experience changes in appetite or dietary habits, leading to nutritional imbalances. Poor nutrition and deficiencies in essential vitamins and minerals can impact hair health. Proper nutrition, including a balanced diet rich in nutrients essential for hair growth, is vital for overall well-being, including hair health.

It is essential to note that while some individuals may experience hair shedding or changes in hair health following a COVID-19 infection, not everyone will be affected in the same way. The severity and duration of hair-related issues may vary among individuals, depending on various factors such as the severity of the infection, individual health status, and underlying conditions.

While experiencing hair changes after a COVID-19 infection can be distressing, it is important to remember that hair issues related to the infection are often temporary and should improve as the body recovers. It is crucial to focus on overall well-being, including mental health, nutrition, and self-care, during the recovery period.

Emotional Eating and Coping Mechanisms

Coping mechanisms are strategies or behaviours individuals adopt to manage and deal with emotional distress or stress. Emotional eating is one such coping mechanism that involves using food as a means of comfort or distraction from negative emotions. While it may provide temporary relief, emotional eating can have negative consequences for both mental and physical well-being, including hair health.

Emotional eating can potentially have an indirect impact on hair health. When individuals engage in emotional eating, they often turn to comfort foods that are typically high in sugar, unhealthy fats, and processed ingredients. These types of foods may lack the essential nutrients necessary for maintaining optimal hair health.

Emotional eating, especially when focused on unhealthy food choices, may lead to a deficiency in the essential nutrients required for healthy hair growth. A diet lacking in adequate protein, vitamins and minerals can contribute to hair loss, brittle hair, slow hair growth and a dull appearance.

Emotional eating in the context of hair issues can arise due to a variety of reasons:

- **Body image concerns:** Hair plays a significant role in our appearance and self-perception. When individuals experience hair issues such as thinning, hair loss, or a change in hair texture, it can lead to dissatisfaction with their appearance and a negative impact on self-esteem. Emotional eating may serve as a temporary coping mechanism to alleviate distress and boost mood.
- **Stress and emotional distress:** Dealing with hair issues can be emotionally challenging, causing stress, anxiety, and frustration. Emotional eating can provide a sense of comfort and distraction from these negative emotions. Food, particularly high-calorie or sugary options, can trigger the release of dopamine (a feel-good neurotransmitter) in the brain, temporarily improving mood.

How to address emotional eating related to hair issues

1. **Recognize triggers**: Pay attention to the specific situations or emotions that lead to emotional eating episodes related to hair concerns. Identifying triggers can help you become more aware of the patterns and develop alternative coping mechanisms.
2. **Seek support:** Share your feelings and concerns with a trusted friend, family member or support group. Talking about your hair issues and receiving support and understanding can provide a sense of relief and help you process your emotions in healthier ways.
3. **Practise self-care:** Engage in activities that promote self-care and boost your overall well-being. This can include activities like exercise, meditation, taking relaxing baths, practising mindfulness or engaging in hobbies that bring you joy and help manage stress.
4. **Seek professional help**: If your hair issues are causing significant distress and affecting your mental and emotional well-being, consider seeking professional help from a therapist or counsellor. They can provide guidance and support to help you navigate through these challenges and develop effective coping strategies.
5. **Focus on overall health:** Instead of resorting to emotional eating, prioritize nourishing your body with a well-balanced, nutrient-rich diet that supports hair health. Ensure you're consuming adequate protein, vitamins, minerals and healthy fats.

Consult with a healthcare professional or a registered dietitian for personalized advice and recommendations.

Affirmations that help!

Our hair plays a significant role in shaping our self-image and overall confidence. However, for some individuals, the mere thought of their hair can trigger negative emotions and affect their mental well-being. If you find yourself in this situation, it's important to focus on promoting hair health while fostering a positive mindset. By incorporating affirmations into your daily routine, you can transform your perspective and cultivate a deep sense of self-acceptance and appreciation. These affirmations serve as powerful reminders that your hair is a unique and beautiful part of you, deserving of love and care.

- ☐ I am grateful for my hair and the role it plays in my unique beauty and identity.
- ☐ My hair is strong, vibrant and resilient, reflecting my overall health and inner strength.
- ☐ I choose to release any negative thoughts or worries about my hair, embracing self-acceptance and love.
- ☐ Each day, I nourish my hair with care, healthy practices and positive energy, supporting its optimal growth and vitality.
- ☐ I am confident in my hair's natural beauty, and I celebrate its uniqueness as a reflection of my individuality.

Summary

Remember, your hair is an integral part of your identity and individuality. By practising affirmations focused on hair health, you are nurturing a positive relationship with your hair, which in turn positively impacts your mental health. Embrace gratitude, release negative thoughts, and nourish your hair with love and care. With time and consistent practice, you'll develop a stronger sense of self-acceptance, allowing you to fully appreciate the beauty and uniqueness of your hair. Embrace the power of positive affirmations and let them guide you on a journey towards healthier hair and a more confident and contented self.

CHAPTER 6

CAN GENES DECIDE THE HEALTH OF YOUR HAIR?

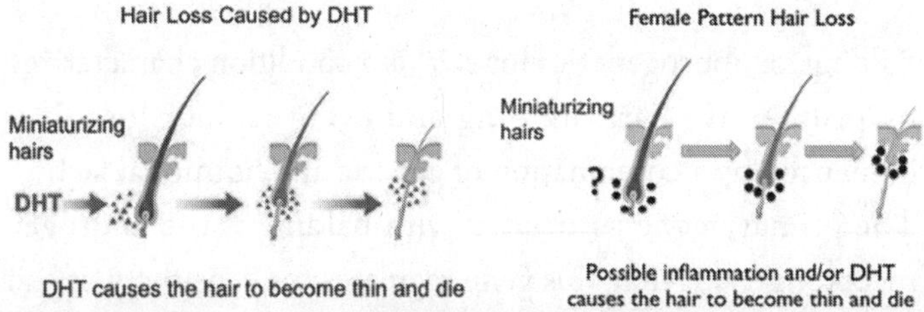

Genes play a big role in determining our hair's texture, whether it's straight, wavy, or curly. They also influence how thick or thin our hair strands are. Scientists have identified specific genes that are linked to these characteristics, and variations in these genes can be associated with different hair textures and thicknesses in people from different ethnic backgrounds.

Sometimes, certain genetic syndromes can cause unusual hair textures. These syndromes involve changes in genes that affect special structures called desmosomes, which help hold hair cells together. Problems with proteins called keratins, which give strength and flexibility to our hair, can also lead to different textures. There are also chemical signals in our bodies, like one called lysophosphatidic acid (LPA), that help promote hair growth, and changes in these signals can be connected to these genetic syndromes.

Understanding the genetic basis of our hair texture and thickness is not only interesting scientifically but also helpful for individuals who want to understand their own hair better. By knowing how genes influence our hair traits, we can appreciate and embrace the natural diversity and beauty of our hair.

Balding:

Balding, or androgenetic alopecia, is a condition characterized by progressive hair thinning and eventual hair loss. It is influenced by a combination of genetic and hormonal factors. The primary gene associated with balding is the androgen receptor gene (AR). This gene regulates the sensitivity of hair follicles to hormones like dihydrotestosterone (DHT), which is derived from testosterone. Individuals with a particular variant of the AR gene may have hair follicles that are more susceptible to the effects of DHT. When DHT binds to the receptors on these hair follicles, it can lead to a process called miniaturization, where the hair follicles shrink in size over time. This miniaturization eventually results in the production of finer and shorter hair strands, leading to visible hair thinning and, ultimately, balding.

Hair Fall:

Excessive hairfall can occur due to various factors, including genetic predisposition. One of the genes associated with hairfall is the transforming growth factor-beta 1 (TGFB1) gene. This gene is involved in regulating the hair growth cycle. Variations or alterations in the TGFB1 gene can disrupt the normal hair growth cycle, leading to increased hair shedding. Additionally, genetic factors related to hormone synthesis and metabolism may also contribute to hairfall. Imbalances in hormones such as oestrogen, testosterone, and thyroid hormones can affect the hair growth cycle and lead to increased hair loss.

Dry Hair:

The moisture content and texture of your hair are influenced by several genes involved in hair shaft structure and moisture retention. Genes encoding keratin proteins, which are the main structural proteins of hair, play a crucial role in determining the strength and elasticity of your hair. Variations in these genes can impact the hair's ability to retain moisture, resulting in dry and brittle hair. Additionally, genes associated with sebum production and lipid metabolism can influence the natural oiliness of the scalp. Sebum, the oil produced by the scalp, helps to lubricate and moisturize the hair. Genetic variations in these genes can affect sebum production, leading to imbalances in scalp and hair moisture levels and contributing to dryness.

Frizzy Hair:

Frizzy hair is often characterized by a lack of moisture and a raised cuticle layer, resulting in unruly and flyaway hair strands. Several genes are involved in determining hair shape and texture. These genes encode proteins such as trichohyalin, keratin-associated proteins and hair follicle receptors. Variations in these genes can affect the structure and arrangement of hair fibres. For example, variations in keratin-associated proteins can alter the bonding and alignment of hair strands, making them more prone to frizz. Additionally, environmental factors like humidity can exacerbate frizz in individuals who are genetically predisposed to it. High humidity causes hair to absorb moisture from the air, leading to swelling of the hair shaft and increased frizz.

What a Nutrigenomic Test Can Do for Your Hair

A nutrigenomic test focuses on how your genes interact with nutrition, providing insights into how your genetic makeup affects your body's response to different nutrients and diets. While it doesn't directly address hair issues, it can be relevant for overall hair health. Here's why:

1. **Nutrient deficiencies:** Nutrients are crucial for healthy hair. A nutrigenomic test can identify genetic variations that affect how your body absorbs and uses essential nutrients for hair health, like vitamins and minerals. With this knowledge, you can adjust your diet or consider targeted supplements to address potential deficiencies.
2. **Inflammation and oxidative stress:** Inflammation and oxidative stress can contribute to hair problems.

Nutrigenomic testing reveals genetic markers related to these processes, helping you understand if you're genetically more prone to inflammation or oxidative damage. Armed with this information, you can choose foods rich in anti-inflammatory and antioxidant properties to support overall hair health.

3. **Nutritional requirements:** Nutrigenomic testing provides insights into your individual nutritional needs based on genetic variations. This helps you make informed dietary choices, like choosing the right balance of macronutrients and specific nutrients that promote hair health. For example, some genetic variations may increase your need for specific vitamins or minerals important for hair growth and maintenance.
4. **Dietary sensitivities:** Genetic variations can affect how your body responds to certain foods. Nutrigenomic testing may uncover potential dietary sensitivities or intolerances that indirectly impact hair health. By avoiding or minimizing these triggers, you can support your overall well-being, including your hair health.

How personalized dietary recommendations based on nutrigenomic testing can optimize nutrient intake for improved hair health?

DNA-based diets have the potential to revolutionize the approach to improving hair health. By analyzing an individual's genetic information, we can gain unique insights into their genetic variations related to nutrient metabolism and utilization. This allows us to design a diet specifically tailored to their genetic profile, optimizing nutrient intake for enhanced hair health.

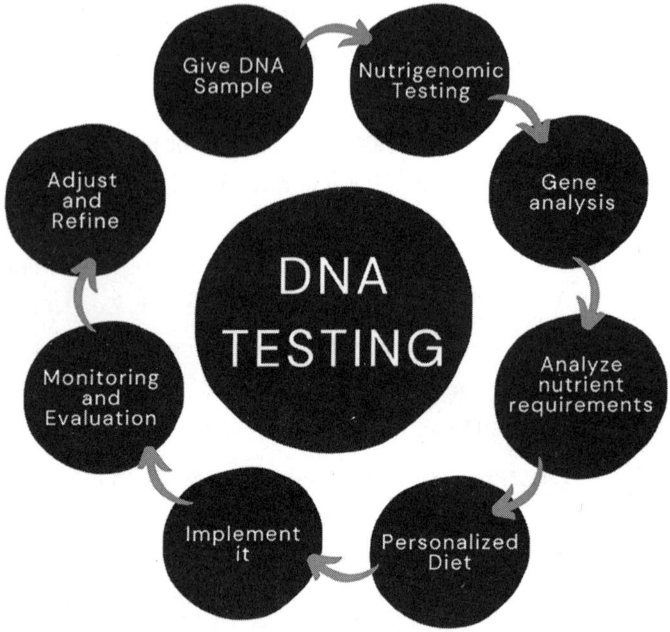

By identifying specific genetic variations, DNA-based diets can address nutrient deficiencies that may affect hair health. These genetic variations can impact the absorption, metabolism, and utilization of key nutrients necessary for hair growth and maintenance. With a DNA-based diet, individuals can ensure they are getting adequate amounts of nutrients such as vitamins, minerals and essential fatty acids to support healthy and vibrant hair.

Moreover, DNA-based diets can help identify food sensitivities or intolerances that may indirectly affect hair health.

Genetic variations can influence an individual's response to certain foods, potentially leading to inflammation or adverse reactions that can impact the condition of their hair. By considering these genetic factors, a DNA-based diet can guide individuals in making informed choices to avoid or minimize the consumption of foods that may negatively affect their hair health.

Genetic variations related to nutrient metabolism and their potential impact on hair health outcomes:

1. **MTHFR gene:** Variations in the MTHFR gene can affect the body's ability to metabolize and utilize folate, an essential nutrient for cell growth and repair. Insufficient folate levels may compromise the health and growth of hair follicles, potentially leading to hair thinning or slow hair growth.
2. **Vitamin D receptor (VDR) gene:** Genetic variations in the VDR gene can influence how the body responds to vitamin D, a nutrient important for hair follicle health. Altered vitamin D metabolism and utilization may contribute to hair loss or impaired hair growth.
3. **Iron metabolism genes:** Genetic variations in genes involved in iron metabolism, such as the HFE gene, can impact the body's ability to absorb and utilize iron. Iron deficiency is a common cause of hair loss, and individuals with certain genetic variations may have a higher risk of developing iron-related hair health issues.
4. **Biotinidase deficiency:** Biotinidase is an enzyme that helps the body convert dietary biotin into a usable form.

Genetic variations in the biotinidase gene can result in biotinidase deficiency, leading to inadequate biotin levels. Biotin is essential for healthy hair growth, and deficiencies may result in brittle hair or hair loss.

5. **Omega-3 fatty acid metabolism genes:** Genetic variations in genes involved in omega-3 fatty acid metabolism, such as FADS1 and FADS2, can affect the body's ability to convert plant-based omega-3 fatty acids into more beneficial forms like EPA and DHA. Omega-3 fatty acids are important for scalp health and may play a role in promoting healthy hair growth.

Gene	Function	Impact on Hair Health
MTHFR	Metabolizes folate	Insufficient levels may lead to hair thinning
VDR	Influences vitamin D response	Altered metabolism may contribute to hair loss
Iron metabolism genes	Regulate iron absorption	Variations can affect iron-related hair issues
Biotinidase	Converts biotin into usable form	Deficiency may lead to brittle hair or hair loss
Omega-3 fatty acid metabolism genes	Metabolize omega-3 fatty acids	Variations can impact scalp health and hair growth

Specific dietary components to add to your DNA-based diet:

- **Collagen**

Collagen is a crucial protein that provides structural support and strength to various tissues in the body, including the hair strands. It is made up of amino acids, which are the building blocks of proteins. Genetic variations related to collagen metabolism can impact the body's ability to produce and maintain healthy collagen levels, which can have implications for hair health.

Collagen deficiencies or imbalances can lead to weaker hair strands, increased brittleness, and a higher susceptibility to damage and breakage.

To optimize collagen production for healthy hair, it is beneficial to include foods rich in collagen-building nutrients in your DNA-based diet. These nutrients provide the necessary amino acids and cofactors for collagen synthesis. Incorporating foods such as bone broth, which is rich in collagen and other supportive nutrients, can provide a natural source of collagen for the body. Additionally, including protein-rich foods like fish, lean meats, poultry, eggs, beans and lentils ensures an adequate intake of amino acids required for collagen production. These dietary sources contribute to the formation of strong and resilient hair strands.

In addition to dietary sources, collagen supplements are available in various forms, including powders and capsules. These supplements can be a convenient way to boost collagen levels in the body, supporting hair health. Collagen supplements are often derived from animal sources, such as fish or bovine collagen, and contain specific types of collagen that are beneficial for hair and overall skin health. It's important to note that while supplements can be a helpful addition, they should be taken under the guidance of a healthcare professional to ensure proper dosage and suitability for individual needs.

- **Vitamin E**

Vitamin E is a key player when it comes to promoting healthy hair, and its effects extend to the genetic level. Your hair-related genes, which are responsible for determining various hair characteristics, can be influenced by vitamin E in multiple ways.

Firstly, vitamin E acts as a powerful antioxidant, safeguarding your hair follicles from oxidative stress. Oxidative stress can damage the DNA within your hair cells, potentially leading to hair problems such as breakage, thinning, and even hair loss. By neutralizing harmful free radicals, vitamin E helps protect the integrity of your hair-related genes, maintaining their optimal function and supporting healthy hair growth.

Moreover, vitamin E plays a role in gene expression, which refers to the activation or suppression of specific genes. Research has shown that vitamin E can modulate the expression of genes involved in hair growth, hair follicle development, and maintenance. By influencing gene expression, vitamin E promotes an environment conducive to healthy hair, helping to ensure that the right genes are activated to support robust hair growth and minimize hair-related issues.

Additionally, studies have highlighted the connection between vitamin E and genes involved in hormone metabolism.

Hormonal imbalances, such as excessive dihydrotestosterone (DHT), can contribute to hair loss. Vitamin E can help regulate hormone metabolism, potentially mitigating the impact of hormonal imbalances on your hair health. This interplay between vitamin E and hair-related genes involved in hormone metabolism underscores the importance of this nutrient in maintaining a healthy hormonal balance and promoting optimal hair growth.

So, by incorporating vitamin E-rich foods into your diet, such as nuts, seeds, spinach, and avocados, you're not only providing your body with an essential nutrient but also supporting your hair-related genes. Remember, each individual's genetic makeup is unique, so consulting with a nutritionist or healthcare professional can provide personalized guidance on incorporating vitamin E and other beneficial nutrients into your DNA-based diet to optimize your hair health.

Case Study: 2

Client Profile	
Age	38 years
Gender	Male

Medical Complications	
Existing Conditions	High blood pressure, fatigue and tiredness
Hair-related Concern	Significant hair loss and male-pattern baldness

DNA Testing Results

Genetic Marker	Gene Name	Result
B12 Capacity	MTHFR	Reduced capacity
B6 Capacity	PDXK	Reduced capacity
PUFA Capacity	PDXK	Reduced capacity
Gluten Intolerance	HLA-DQ2/DQ8	Present
Alopecia Risk	KRTAP1-1	Moderate

Existing Diet and Exercise	
Diet	He follows a well-balanced and nutritious diet, incorporating plenty of fresh fruits, vegetables, lean proteins, and whole grains. His diet is rich in essential vitamins and minerals, providing the necessary nutrients for overall health, including hair health.
Exercise	He maintains an active lifestyle to counteract the sedentary nature of his occupation. He dedicates time every morning to engaging in rigorous workouts, which may include cardio exercises, weightlifting, or high-intensity interval training. Additionally, he enjoys taking walks in the evenings to unwind and further promote physical activity. Despite his healthy diet and regular exercise, he experiences

	physical strain due to stress from work and other factors, which can potentially impact his overall health, including his hair health.

Recommendations and Intervention	
Gut Health Improvement	Incorporate probiotic-rich foods into the diet. Consider a probiotic supplement.
Lifestyle Modifications	Encourage regular physical activity and exercise. Modify the workout routine based on the client's DNA report. Since ABC is a morning person, according to the DNA report, shift the workout sessions to the morning instead of the afternoon. Reduce workout intensity to prevent excessive physical strain.

Improvement in Hair	
Hair Loss Reduction	After four months of following the recommended dietary and lifestyle changes, he observed a significant reduction in hair loss. The frequency and severity of hair shedding continued to decrease, with a noticeable improvement in hair retention.

Scalp Health Improvement	He experienced further improvements in scalp health. The previously itchy scalp and excessive dandruff continued to reduce, indicating a healthier scalp environment. Additionally, thinning areas of the scalp showed continued signs of improvement.
Hair Regrowth	He continued to notice new hair growth in previously sparse areas. The new hair growth appeared to be denser and thicker, contributing to an improved overall hair appearance.
Overall Well-being	In addition to the ongoing improvement in hair health, he reported sustained feelings of increased energy and improved well-being. The positive changes in diet, lifestyle, and hair health continued to positively impact his overall health and confidence.

Summary

In this chapter, we explore the influence of genes on hair health. Genes play a significant role in determining hair texture, thickness, and susceptibility to hair loss. Variations in genes such as MTHFR, VDR, and those related to iron metabolism, biotinidase, and omega-3 fatty acid metabolism can impact nutrient absorption, hormone response, and overall hair health.

Understanding the genetic basis of hair traits can help individuals embrace the natural diversity of their hair and make informed choices for optimal haircare. Nutrigenomic testing can further optimize nutrient intake for improved hair health by identifying individual nutritional needs based on genetic variations. By incorporating personalized dietary recommendations based on nutrigenomic testing, individuals can address nutrient deficiencies, support scalp and hair health, and optimize overall hair well-being.

CHAPTER 7

HYDRATION FOR HEALTHY HAIR

Believe it or not, water makes up almost 25 per cent of the weight of a single strand of hair.

Hydration is crucial for maintaining the health and vitality of your hair. It starts with your scalp, which serves as the foundation for strong and beautiful hair. When you apply hydrating products or oils, they penetrate deep into the hair follicles, nourishing the living cells in the hair shaft. This ensures that your hair receives the oxygen, water and nutrients it needs to grow and thrive.

Proper hydration is the key to keeping your hair resilient and preventing dryness and brittleness. By maintaining adequate moisture levels, you can preserve the elasticity and strength of your hair, reducing the risk of breakage and maintaining a vibrant appearance.

In addition to hydration, your hair products are enriched with essential vitamins and minerals. These nutrients not only nourish your hair during application but also help to retain moisture even after washing. This means that your hair receives ongoing hydration and remains soft, manageable and full of life.

Transporting Nutrients to Hair

When it comes to haircare, hydration takes centre stage as the essential element for maintaining healthy locks. But hydration does more than just moisturize your hair; it plays a crucial role in transporting vital nutrients to your scalp, laying the foundation for strong and vibrant hair growth.

Your scalp is home to a higher concentration of sebaceous glands, which are responsible for secreting oils that provide moisture and nourishment to your hair follicles, preventing dryness and promoting a healthy scalp environment. However, for these oils to effectively reach the follicles, they need the assistance of hydration.

Water acts as the ultimate transporter, facilitating the flow of nutrients to your scalp through tiny blood vessels called capillaries. These capillaries are strategically located near each hair follicle, ensuring that oxygen and nutrients from various parts of your body, including your heart and lungs, reach your scalp and get absorbed by the hair follicles.

But hydration's role doesn't end there. Water also promotes the production of collagen and elastin at the root tip, strengthening the hair fibres and preventing breakage. By staying properly hydrated, you provide the necessary building blocks for strong, resilient hair. On the flip side, dehydration can negatively impact both the quality and growth of your hair. You may have noticed that your hair tends to get dry during certain times of the year, especially in the summer. The culprit is inadequate water intake. When you don't drink enough water, your hair is left thirsting for moisture, leading to dryness and lackluster locks.

So, remember to keep yourself hydrated throughout the day, ensuring that your hair receives the nutrients it needs to thrive. Your hair will thank you with its shine, strength, and overall vitality. Cheers to nourishing your hair from within!

Water plays a vital role in haircare, as it acts as a carrier for essential nutrients and promotes overall hair health.

Here's a closer look at the role of water in haircare and its function as a nutrient:

- **Hydration and moisture:** Water is essential for maintaining optimal hydration and moisture in your hair. Each hair strand consists of multiple layers, and the outermost layer, known as the cuticle, acts as a protective barrier. When your hair is well-hydrated, the cuticle lies flat, allowing it to retain moisture effectively. This helps to prevent dryness, brittleness and frizz, giving your hair a smoother and healthier appearance.

  Water molecules penetrate the hair shaft, helping to replenish and maintain the moisture balance within the hair. When the hair strands lack moisture, they can become dry, brittle, and more susceptible to breakage. Hydrated hair, on the other hand, retains its elasticity, making it more resistant to damage and reducing the likelihood of breakage and split ends. It also enhances the manageability of your hair, making it easier to style and reducing tangles.

Furthermore, well-hydrated hair is less prone to frizz. When your hair lacks moisture, it tends to absorb moisture from the environment, causing the cuticle to swell and the hair strands to become frizzy. By keeping your hair properly hydrated, you create a protective barrier that prevents excessive moisture absorption, helping to control frizz and maintain a smoother and more polished look.

- **Nutrient transport:** Water acts as a carrier for essential nutrients, vitamins and minerals, facilitating their transportation to the scalp and hair follicles. These nutrients are crucial for nourishing the hair follicles, promoting healthy hair growth, and maintaining the overall health of your hair.
- **Scalp health:** Adequate water intake is necessary for maintaining a well-hydrated scalp. A hydrated scalp promotes the proper functioning of the sebaceous glands, which produce natural oils that keep the scalp moisturized and nourished. This helps to prevent dry scalp conditions, dandruff and itchiness.
- **Oxygen supply:** Water is also important for delivering oxygen to the hair follicles through the bloodstream. Oxygen is essential for cellular respiration and the metabolic processes that support hair growth. Sufficient oxygen supply to the hair follicles promotes healthier, stronger and more vibrant hair.

- **Hair elasticity and strength:** Water contributes to the elasticity and strength of the hair strands. Proper hydration allows the hair to maintain its natural elasticity, making it more resilient to damage and reducing the likelihood of breakage. Hydrated hair is less prone to split ends and maintains its integrity and shine.

Internal Hydration vs External Hydration:

When it comes to keeping our hair hydrated, we often hear about the importance of both internal and external hydration. But what exactly do these terms mean, and how do they differ? Let's take a closer look at internal and external hydration and their roles in maintaining healthy, hydrated hair.

Internal Hydration

Internal hydration refers to the process of nourishing our bodies with fluids by consuming an adequate amount of water and other hydrating beverages. It is the foundation of long-term hair health, as it directly affects the overall hydration and health of our hair strands and follicles.

Drinking enough water is essential for the proper functioning of our body systems, and our hair follicles are no exception. When we consume an adequate amount of water, it circulates through our bloodstream, reaching the hair follicles and nourishing them from within. This internal hydration helps maintain the moisture balance in our hair strands, keeping them hydrated, supple and resilient.

Proper internal hydration ensures that our hair follicles receive the necessary nutrients and oxygen, promoting healthy hair growth and preventing dryness and brittleness. It also supports the overall health of our scalp, preventing dry scalp conditions and enhancing the optimal environment for hair growth.

To maintain internal hydration, it is recommended to drink an adequate amount of water throughout the day. While individual water needs may vary based on factors such as body weight, activity level, and climate, aiming for about eight glasses (64 ounces) of water per day is a good start. Remember, staying hydrated from within provides a solid foundation for maintaining healthy, hydrated hair.

External Hydration

External hydration involves using moisturizing hair products to provide a temporary boost of moisture to the hair strands. These products, such as conditioners, hair masks, and leave-in treatments, work by creating a barrier that seals in moisture and helps prevent water loss from the hair.

While external hydration can improve the immediate moisture content of the hair, its effects are often temporary. Without proper internal hydration, the benefits of external hydration can be short-lived. Think of external hydration as a supplemental measure to support the overall health and hydration of the hair, rather than a standalone solution.

Moisturizing hair products can be beneficial for maintaining hair moisture, enhancing manageability, and improving the appearance of dry or damaged hair. They help to smooth the hair cuticles, reducing frizz and improving shine. However, it's important to note that relying solely on external hydration without prioritizing internal hydration may lead to incomplete and temporary results.

To make the most of external hydration, incorporate it as part of a holistic haircare routine that includes both internal and external hydration. By ensuring proper internal hydration, you provide a solid foundation for your hair to absorb and retain moisture from external sources effectively.

	Internal Hydration for Hair	**External Hydration for Hair**
Definition	Nourishing the hair from within by consuming fluids	Applying moisturizing hair products externally to improve moisture content
Role	Maintains overall hair health and hydration by providing nutrients to the hair follicles	Provides a temporary moisture boost and improves the immediate appearance of hair
Benefits	Ensures long-term hair health, hydration and growth	Enhances hair moisture, manageability and appearance temporarily

	Internal Hydration for Hair	External Hydration for Hair
Method	Consuming an adequate amount of water and hydrating beverages	Using conditioners, hair masks and leave-in treatments to seal in moisture
Duration	Continuous and ongoing as part of a healthy lifestyle	Temporary effects until the next wash or application of hair products
Importance	Provides a solid foundation for maintaining healthy, hydrated hair	Complements internal hydration and supports moisture retention in the hair
Key Focus	Nourishing the hair follicles, preventing dryness and brittleness	Improving moisture balance, reducing frizz, and enhancing shine

Summary

Hydration is a crucial factor in maintaining healthy and vibrant hair. Water plays a vital role in haircare as it acts as a carrier for essential nutrients, promotes moisture balance, and supports overall hair health. Proper internal hydration, achieved through consuming an adequate amount of water, nourishes the hair follicles from within, ensuring long-term hair health, growth, and hydration. On the other hand, external hydration, through the use of moisturizing hair products, provides a temporary moisture boost and improves the immediate appearance of the hair. While external hydration is beneficial, it is important to prioritize internal hydration as it forms the foundation for maintaining healthy, hydrated hair. By combining both internal and external hydration approaches, we can achieve optimal hair hydration, strength, and vitality.

CHAPTER 8

ESSENTIAL NUTRIENTS FOR HAIRCARE

When it comes to achieving long, thick and beautiful hair, various factors come into play. Genetics, age, and environmental influences all play a role in determining the quality of our hair. However, there's one undeniable truth: the appearance of your hair reflects what you feed your body. Our bodies are incredibly intelligent, prioritizing essential organs and vital functions over non-essential ones like hair and nails. While we may cherish our luscious locks, our bodies have other priorities. This understanding emphasizes the importance of nourishing our bodies with optimal nutrition to support healthy hair, as well as skin and nails.

To ensure your hair thrives, it all starts with a nutrient-dense diet that provides enough energy (calories) based on your age and activity level. Highly processed foods might be calorie-dense, but they often lack essential nutrients. Instead, focusing on real, whole foods—the ones that require cutting, cooking, and preparation—will nourish not only your body but also your hair. By embracing a variety of wholesome foods, you and your

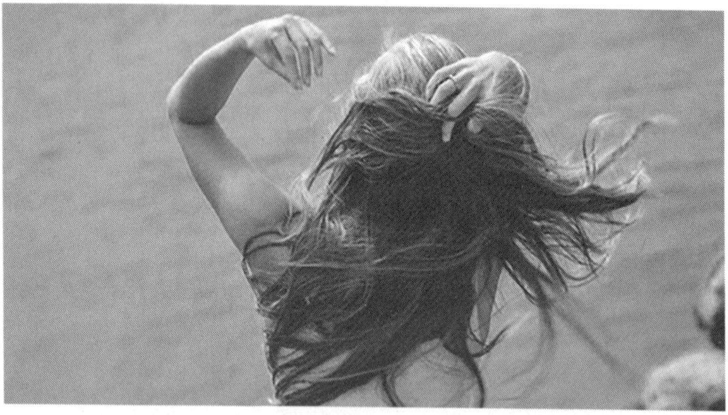

hair will reap the benefits of vibrant health and vitality. So, let's embark on a journey to nurture ourselves from within, radiating that beauty through our hair and beyond.

If you want to go a step further, make a point of prioritizing the 13 nutrients below.

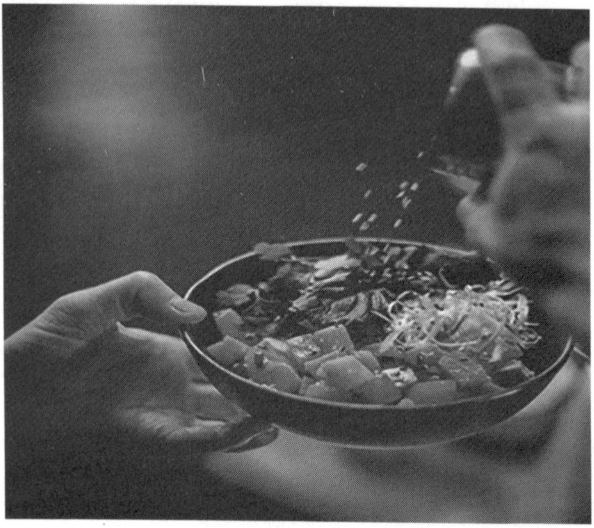

Protein

Your hair is made from protein, so it stands to reason that protein plays a crucial role in how strong and healthy it is. Eating a diet too low in protein can lead to dry, brittle hair and even hair loss. Nuts, seeds, legumes, meat and fish are all good sources of protein. Collagen protein is particularly helpful in the formation and strengthening of your hair. Protein not only contributes to the overall health of your hair but also helps to reduce hair porosity.

Porous hair has non-uniform gaps that make it susceptible to damage from external elements like colours and pollutants, which can easily get absorbed into the gaps. Adequate protein levels in your hair can protect it from various side effects of chemicals that may be present in hair dyes. Furthermore, protein acts as the building block of your hair and plays a vital role in restoring damaged hair tissues, ensuring durability and fullness. With the right protein levels in your hair, you can enjoy thick, shiny and bouncy locks. In maintaining the health, strength, and appearance of our hair, protein plays a crucial role. Hair is primarily composed of a protein called keratin, and consuming an adequate amount of protein is essential for its growth, repair and overall health.

Protein is made up of amino acids, the building blocks of our body. When we consume protein-rich foods, our body breaks them down into amino acids and uses them to build and repair various tissues, including the hair follicles. So, next time you enjoy a protein-packed meal, know that you're not only nourishing your body but also giving your hair the foundation it needs to look and feel its best.

(i) What does low protein intake lead to?

Protein deficiency can have a significant impact on hair quality. Insufficient protein intake can lead to hair thinning, hair loss and weakened hair strands. This occurs because when our body is lacking in protein, it prioritizes other essential functions over hair growth. As a result, the hair follicles enter a resting phase known as the telogen phase, which leads to increased shedding and reduced hair growth.

(ii) What is the recommended dosage of protein?

The recommended daily intake of protein varies depending on factors such as age, sex, weight, and activity level. However, as a general guideline, adults should aim for around 0.8 grams of protein per kilogram of body weight. For example, if you weigh 60 kilograms, you would need approximately 48 grams of protein per day. However, individuals with specific health conditions or higher physical activity levels may require more protein.

(iii) What are the best vegetarian and non-vegetarian sources of protein?

Both vegetarian and non-vegetarian sources provide protein that can benefit hair health.

Vegetarian Sources:

→ Legumes: Lentils, chickpeas, black beans and kidney beans

→ Nuts and seeds: Almonds, walnuts, chia seeds, flaxseeds and hemp seeds

→ Wholegrains: Quinoa (A pseudo-grain that is a complete protein source, meaning it contains all nine essential amino acids.)

→ Tofu and tempeh: Soy-based products that are protein-rich and suitable for vegetarians and vegans

Non-vegetarian Sources:

→ Lean meats: Chicken breast, turkey breast and lean cuts of pork

→ Fish and seafood: Salmon, tuna, shrimp and other seafood varieties

→ Eggs: One large egg contains approximately 6 grams of protein and is a versatile option for incorporating protein into your diet.

B Vitamins

The B vitamins form a vital family of nutrients, and many of them play a significant role in maintaining strong and healthy hair. These essential vitamins are responsible for enhancing blood circulation to the scalp, stimulating hair follicles, and promoting the growth of lustrous hair. Moreover, they are instrumental in reducing hair loss and contributing to longer, shinier locks.

Several B vitamins are particularly beneficial for hair health. B2 (riboflavin), niacin, pantothenic acid, folic acid, B6, and

B12 are all known to support strong and vibrant hair. Among them, biotin deserves special mention as it actively stimulates the growth of new cells. Together, these B vitamins are often referred to as vitamin B complexes, and they play a significant role in maintaining overall health. Their impact reaches far beyond hair health, as they also influence energy levels, metabolism, nerves, muscles, skin, nails, and overall well-being.

The B vitamin complex collectively promotes cell growth and division, which is crucial for the healthy growth of hair. It's essential to replenish your body's supply of these water-soluble vitamins daily, as they cannot be stored in the body. Any excess amounts that the body doesn't use are flushed out through urine. Among the B vitamins, niacin stands out for its role in nourishing the scalp and promoting healthy hair growth.

(i) What does low B vitamins intake lead to?

Insufficient amounts of niacin can lead to brittle and lifeless hair and even hair loss. So, ensure you include a variety of B vitamin-rich foods in your daily diet to support not only your overall health but also the strength and vibrancy of your hair. With the proper intake of these essential nutrients, you can take great strides towards maintaining gorgeous and resilient locks.

(ii) What is the recommended dosage of B vitamins?

The recommended dosage of B vitamins can vary depending on factors such as age, sex, individual health needs and the specific B vitamins in question. Here are the general recommended dietary allowances (RDAs) for the different B vitamins:

Vitamin B1 (thiamine):

→ Adult men: 1.2 mg per day

→ Adult women: 1.1 mg per day

Vitamin B2 (riboflavin):

→ Adult men: 1.3 mg per day

→ Adult women: 1.1 mg per day

Vitamin B3 (niacin):

→ Adult men: 16 mg NE (niacin equivalents) per day

→ Adult women: 14 mg NE per day

Vitamin B5 (pantothenic acid):

→ The adequate intake for adults is typically 5 mg per day.

Vitamin B6 (pyridoxine):

→ Adult men: 1.3 to 1.7 mg per day, depending on age

→ Adult women: 1.3 to 1.5 mg per day, depending on age

Vitamin B7 (biotin):

→ The adequate intake for adults is typically 30 mcg (micrograms) per day.

Vitamin B9 (folic acid or folate):

→ Adult men and women: 400 mcg per day

→ Pregnant women: 600 mcg per day

Vitamin B12 (cobalamin):

→ Adult men and women: 2.4 mcg per day

(iii) What are the best vegetarian and non-vegetarian sources for B vitamins?

Here are some of the best sources of B vitamins for both vegetarians and non-vegetarians:

Vegetarian Sources

Vitamin B1 (thiamine):

- Whole grains (brown rice, oats and quinoa)
- Legumes (black beans, lentils and chickpeas)
- Nuts and seeds (sunflower seeds and flaxseeds)
- Fortified cereals

Vitamin B2 (riboflavin):

- Dairy products (milk and yoghurt)
- Fortified plant-based milk (almond milk and soy milk)
- Leafy green vegetables (spinach and kale)
- Mushrooms

Vitamin B3 (niacin):

- Legumes (peanuts and peas)
- Whole grains (brown rice and whole wheat)

Vitamin B5 (pantothenic acid):

- Avocado
- Whole grains (oats and brown rice)
- Legumes (chickpeas and lentils)

Vitamin B6 (pyridoxine):

- Potatoes
- Bananas
- Legumes (lentils and chickpeas)
- Nuts and seeds (sunflower seeds and pistachios)

Vitamin B7 (biotin):

- Nuts and seeds (almonds and peanuts)
- Sweet potatoes
- Spinach

Vitamin B9 (folic acid or folate):

- Leafy green vegetables (spinach and kale)
- Legumes (black beans and lentils)
- Fortified cereals

Non-vegetarian Sources:

Vitamin B1 (thiamine):

- Pork

- Fish (salmon and trout)
- Poultry (chicken and turkey)

Vitamin B2 (riboflavin):

- Organ meats (liver)
- Fish (salmon and mackerel)
- Poultry (chicken)

Vitamin B3 (niacin):

- Poultry (chicken and turkey)
- Fish (tuna and salmon)
- Pork

Vitamin B5 (pantothenic acid):

- Organ meats (liver)
- Poultry (chicken)
- Fish (salmon and trout)

Vitamin B6 (pyridoxine):

- Poultry (chicken and turkey)
- Fish (salmon and tuna)
- Pork

Vitamin B7 (biotin):

- Organ meats (liver)
- Egg yolks

Vitamin B9 (Folic Acid or Folate):

- Organ meats (liver)
- Poultry (chicken and turkey)
- Fish (salmon and trout)

Iron

Iron is an essential mineral for hair health and plays a crucial role in maintaining strong and vibrant hair. Iron is involved in the production of haemoglobin, a protein in red blood cells that carries oxygen from the lungs to various tissues in the body, including the hair follicles. Adequate iron levels ensure that oxygen is efficiently delivered to the hair follicles, promoting healthy hair growth and preventing hair loss. Iron is essential for cell division and the repair of damaged cells, which is essential for the growth and maintenance of healthy hair. Iron deficiency (anaemia) can lead to hair loss as the hair follicles may enter a resting phase due to insufficient oxygen and nutrients. Proper iron levels contribute to the overall texture and strength of the hair, preventing brittleness and breakage.

(i) What does low iron intake lead to?

Low iron intake can lead to hair problems, primarily due to iron's crucial role in the production of haemoglobin, a protein in red blood cells responsible for carrying oxygen to various tissues, including the hair follicles. When the body doesn't receive enough iron through the diet, it can lead to iron deficiency or anaemia, which can have adverse effects on hair health.

Iron deficiency can lead to a condition called telogen effluvium, where a large number of hair follicles enter a resting phase prematurely, causing increased hair shedding. This can result in noticeable hair thinning and hair loss.

Insufficient iron levels can affect the hair's growth cycle, leading to slower hair growth and reduced hair density. Low iron levels can weaken the hair structure, making it brittle and more prone to breakage. Lack of iron can lead to reduced oxygen supply to the hair follicles, resulting in dull, lacklustre and lifeless hair. In some cases, iron deficiency may alter the hair's texture, making it dry and coarse.

(ii) What is the recommended dosage of iron?

The recommended daily intake of iron varies depending on factors such as age, sex, and life stage.

The following are the general recommended dietary allowances (RDAs) for iron:

- Infants (0–6 months): 0.27 mg
- Infants (7–12 months): 11 mg
- Children (1–3 years): 7 mg
- Children (4–8 years): 10 mg
- Males (9–13 years): 8 mg
- Females (9–13 years): 8 mg
- Males (14–18 years): 11 mg
- Females (14–18 years): 15 mg
- Adult males (19–50 years): 8 mg

- → Adult females (19–50 years): 18 mg (due to menstrual losses)
- → Pregnant females: 27 mg
- → Breastfeeding females: 9–10 mg

(iii) What are the best vegetarian and non-vegetarian sources of iron?

Vegetarian Sources:

- → Legumes: Lentils, chickpeas, kidney beans, black beans and soybeans
- → Nuts and seeds: Pumpkin seeds, sunflower seeds, hemp seeds and almonds
- → Whole grains: Quinoa, oats, fortified cereals and brown rice
- → Leafy green vegetables: Spinach, kale, Swiss chard and collard greens
- → Tofu: Firm tofu is a plant-based source of iron.
- → Fortified plant-based foods: Fortified cereals, bread and plant-based milk

Non-vegetarian Sources:

- → Red meat: Lamb and pork
- → Poultry: Chicken and turkey
- → Fish: Certain fish, such as salmon, tuna and sardines
- → Shellfish: Shrimp, clams and mussels

Tips to Enhance Iron Absorption

- Vitamin C: Consuming vitamin C-rich foods along with iron-rich foods can enhance iron absorption. Citrus fruits, strawberries, bell peppers, and tomatoes are excellent sources of vitamin C.
- Avoid coffee and tea: Coffee and tea contain compounds that can inhibit iron absorption. It's best to avoid consuming them with iron-rich meals.
- Cast-iron cookware: Cooking acidic foods, such as tomatoes or beans, in cast-iron cookware can increase the iron content of the food.
- Calcium consideration: If you take calcium supplements, avoid taking them with iron-rich foods, as calcium can interfere with iron absorption.

Vitamin C

Vitamin C, also known as ascorbic acid, is a crucial nutrient for maintaining healthy hair. It plays several roles in supporting hair growth, strengthening the hair shaft, and promoting overall hair health. Vitamin C is essential for the synthesis of collagen, a protein that provides structure to the hair follicles and promotes hair strength and elasticity.

As an antioxidant, vitamin C protects the hair follicles and scalp from oxidative stress caused by free radicals. It helps to neutralize damaging free radicals and prevent hair cell damage. Vitamin C enhances the absorption of iron from plant-based sources, which is crucial for the transportation of oxygen to the hair follicles. Sufficient iron levels are necessary for healthy hair growth.

(i) What does low vitamin C intake lead to?

Inadequate intake of vitamin C can lead to various hair-related issues. Vitamin C deficiency can contribute to the dryness and brittleness of the hair strands, making them more prone to breakage. Insufficient vitamin C levels can negatively impact hair growth, resulting in slower hair growth or stunted hair follicle development. Vitamin C plays a role in maintaining the strength and integrity of the hair structure. Low levels can lead to weakened hair shafts and increased vulnerability to damage.

(ii) What is the recommended dosage of vitamin C?

The recommended daily intake of vitamin C varies depending on age, sex and life stage.

The following are the general recommended dietary allowances (RDAs) for vitamin C:

- Infants (0–6 months): 40 mg
- Infants (7–12 months): 50 mg
- Children (1–3 years): 15 mg
- Children (4–8 years): 25 mg
- Children (9–13 years): 45 mg
- Adolescent males (14–18 years): 75 mg
- Adolescent females (14–18 years): 65 mg
- Adult males (19 years and older): 90 mg

- → Adult females (19 years and older): 75 mg
- → Pregnant females (18 years and younger): 80 mg
- → Pregnant females (19 years and older): 85 mg
- → Breastfeeding females (18 years and younger): 115 mg
- → Breastfeeding females (19 years and older): 120 mg

(iii) What are the best vegetarian and non-vegetarian sources of vitamin C?

Vegetarian Sources:

- → Citrus fruits: Oranges, lemons, grapefruits and tangerines
- → Berries: Strawberries, blueberries, raspberries and blackberries
- → Kiwi
- → Papaya
- → Guava
- → Pineapple
- → Mango
- → Tomato
- → Bell peppers: Particularly red, yellow and green bell peppers
- → Broccoli
- → Spinach

Non-vegetarian Sources:

→ Meats: Animal-based foods such as pork, chicken, turkey and organ meats like liver

→ Seafood: Fish like salmon and mackerel

Vitamin D

Vitamin D is a crucial nutrient that plays a significant role in hair health. It supports the growth and maintenance of hair follicles, helps prevent hair loss and contributes to overall hair quality. It is involved in various physiological processes that influence hair growth and health. It helps stimulate hair follicles and promotes the production of new hair cells. Adequate levels contribute to strong, healthy hair strands and a well-nourished scalp. Additionally, it supports the immune system, which is essential for maintaining a healthy scalp environment.

(i) What does low vitamin D intake lead to?

Insufficient vitamin D levels can negatively impact hair quality and contribute to hair loss. Low levels of vitamin D have been associated with conditions like alopecia areata, a form of hair loss characterized by patchy bald spots. Vitamin D deficiency may also lead to hair thinning, brittleness and slower hair growth. It is important to maintain optimal vitamin D levels to support healthy hair growth and prevent hair-related issues.

(ii) What is the recommended dosage of vitamin D?

The recommended dosage of vitamin D can vary depending on age, health conditions, and individual needs.

The following are the general guidelines for daily vitamin D intake for most poeple:

For most people

- → Infants (0–12 months): 400–1000 IU (International Units) per day
- → Children (1–18 years): 600–1000 IU per day
- → Adults (19–70 years): 600–800 IU per day
- → Adults (over 70 years): 800–1000 IU per day

For some specific groups

- → Pregnant and breastfeeding women: 600–800 IU per day

Note: The above-recommended dosages are for total vitamin D intake, including both dietary and supplemental sources.

(iii) What are the best vegetarian and non-vegetarian sources of vitamin D?

Vegetarian Sources:

- → Mushrooms: Some mushrooms, particularly wild mushrooms and those exposed to ultraviolet (UV) light, can synthesize vitamin D2.
- → Fortified foods: Certain plant-based foods are fortified with vitamin D2, such as fortified plant-based milk, cheese, yoghurt, orange juice and breakfast cereals.
- → Fortified plant-based milk: Some plant-based milk alternatives, like soy milk, almond milk, and oat milk, are fortified with vitamin D2.

→ Fortified tofu: Certain types of tofu are fortified with vitamin D2.

Non-vegetarian Sources:

Fatty fish are among the best natural sources of vitamin D3, which is the most biologically active form of vitamin D. Examples include:

→ Salmon

→ Mackerel

→ Sardines

→ Trout

→ Herring

→ Cod liver oil is an excellent source of vitamin D3.

→ Egg yolks contain small amounts of vitamin D3.

Vitamin E

Vitamin E, known as tocopherol, is a fat-soluble vitamin with powerful antioxidant properties. It plays a crucial role in maintaining the health and vitality of our hair. Vitamin E improves blood circulation to the scalp, ensuring an adequate supply of oxygen and nutrients. This promotes a healthy scalp environment for hair growth. As an antioxidant, vitamin E neutralizes free radicals that can damage hair follicles and contribute to hair loss or premature greying. Vitamin E helps retain moisture in the hair, reducing dryness, frizz, and brittleness. It adds shine and improves overall hair texture.

(i) What does low vitamin E intake lead to?

Vitamin E levels can impact hair health and lead to various problems. Vitamin E deficiency can cause dryness, dullness and increased susceptibility to breakage. Insufficient vitamin E may disrupt the normal hair growth cycle, resulting in slower hair growth or thinning. Vitamin E deficiency can contribute to a dry, flaky scalp and, in severe cases, may even lead to hair loss.

(ii) What is the recommended dosage of vitamin E?

The recommended dosage of vitamin E can vary depending on age, sex, and life stage.

The following are the general guidelines for daily vitamin E intake, expressed in milligrams (mg) of alpha-tocopherol equivalents (ATE):

For most people,

→ Infants (0–6 months): 4 mg ATE per day
→ Infants (7–12 months): 5 mg ATE per day
→ Children (1–3 years): 6 mg ATE per day
→ Children (4–8 years): 7 mg ATE per day
→ Children (9–13 years): 11 mg ATE per day
→ Adolescents (14–18 years): 15 mg ATE per day
→ Adults (19 years and older): 15 mg ATE per day

For pregnant and breastfeeding women,

- Pregnant and breastfeeding women (under 18 years): 15 mg ATE per day
- Pregnant and breastfeeding women (19 years and older): 19 mg ATE per day

(iii) What are the best vegetarian and non-vegetarian sources of vitamin E?

Vegetarian Sources:

- Nuts and seeds: Almonds, sunflower seeds, hazelnuts and peanuts
- Plant-based oils: Wheat germ oil, sunflower oil, safflower oil and almond oil
- Leafy green vegetables: Spinach, Swiss chard and kale contain vitamin E.
- Avocado
- Fortified cereals: Some breakfast cereals are fortified with vitamin E
- Kiwi

Non-vegetarian Sources:

Some types of fish contain vitamin E, although in lower amounts compared to plant-based sources.

- Rainbow trout
- Salmon

- → Sardines
- → Shellfish: Shrimp and lobster contain small amounts of vitamin E

Vitamin A

Vitamin A is a vital and versatile nutrient that plays a crucial role in supporting various aspects of human health. As a fat-soluble vitamin, it is stored in the body's fat tissues and liver, making it available when needed. Vitamin A is essential for maintaining good vision, promoting a robust immune system, supporting cell growth and differentiation, and contributing to healthy skin and mucous membranes. It is involved in crucial processes ranging from vision in dim light to regulating gene expression and fostering proper growth and development. The oily substance produced by your scalp that keeps your head from becoming dry and itchy and keeps your hair hydrated depends on vitamin A. This natural conditioner is secreted by your sebaceous glands, and without enough vitamin A, we can't produce enough of it.

(i) What does low vitamin A intake lead to?

Low vitamin A intake can lead to a range of health issues and deficiencies, including night blindness, xerophthalmia (dry eyes), impaired immune function, skin problems, reduced growth and development, reproductive issues, and weakened mucous membrane integrity. Vitamin A is crucial for vision, immune system support, cell growth, and healthy skin and mucous membranes.

(ii) What is the recommended dosage of vitamin A?

The recommended daily intake of vitamin A can vary depending on age, sex, and life stage.

The following are the general guidelines for daily vitamin A intake, expressed in micrograms (mcg) of retinol activity equivalents (RAE):

For most people,

- → Infants (0–6 months): 400 mcg RAE per day
- → Infants (7–12 months): 500 mcg RAE per day
- → Children (1–3 years): 300 mcg RAE per day
- → Children (4–8 years): 400 mcg RAE per day
- → Children (9–13 years): 600 mcg RAE per day
- → Adolescents (14–18 years):
    - → Males: 900 mcg RAE per day
    - → Females: 700 mcg RAE per day
- → Adults (19 years and older):
    - → Males: 900 mcg RAE per day
    - → Females: 700 mcg RAE per day

For pregnant and breastfeeding women,

- → Pregnant women: 770–1300 mcg RAE per day, depending on age
- → Breastfeeding women: 1300–1500 mcg RAE per day, depending on age

(iii) What are the best vegetarian and non-vegetarian sources of vitamin A?

Vegetarian Sources:

- → Sweet potatoes
- → Carrots
- → Spinach
- → Kale
- → Mangoes
- → Apricots
- → Pumpkin
- → Cantaloupe
- → Red bell peppers

Non-vegetarian Sources:

- → Liver, particularly beef liver
- → Fish liver oils, such as cod liver oil
- → Salmon
- → Dairy products like milk, cheese and yoghurt

Zinc

Zinc is a vital mineral with diverse roles in the body. It supports the immune system, aids in wound healing, and promotes healthy cell growth and division. Zinc acts as an antioxidant, protects DNA, and influences taste and smell perception. Additionally, it regulates hormones and is crucial for growth and development. In some cases, a dry, flaky scalp can be caused by zinc deficiency. Lack of zinc can also lead to hair loss and acne in some people.

Zinc is involved in DNA and protein synthesis, which are essential for hair growth. It helps regulate cell division and supports the growth of hair follicles. Zinc is necessary for proper hormone production and regulation. Hormonal imbalances can contribute to hair loss or thinning, and zinc helps maintain hormonal balance. Zinc has antimicrobial properties that help keep the scalp healthy and prevent dandruff, itchiness and infections. A healthy scalp provides a favourable environment for hair growth.

(i) What does a low zinc intake lead to?

Low zinc intake can result in impaired immune function, leading to increased vulnerability to infections. It may also cause delayed wound healing and hinder proper growth and development, particularly in children. Zinc deficiency can lead to skin problems, hair loss, and a decreased sense of taste and smell. Inadequate zinc intake or low zinc levels in the body can affect hair quality and contribute to hair problems such as hair loss, thinning, dullness and slow hair growth. Zinc deficiency can disrupt the normal hair growth cycle and lead to weakened hair follicles.

(ii) What is the recommended dosage of zinc?

The recommended daily intake of zinc can vary depending on age, sex, and life stage.

The following are the general guidelines for daily zinc intake, expressed in milligrams (mg):

For most people,

- → Infants (0–6 months): 2 mg per day
- → Infants (7–12 months): 3 mg per day
- → Children (1–3 years): 3 mg per day
- → Children (4–8 years): 5 mg per day
- → Children (9–13 years): 8 mg per day
- → Adolescents (14–18 years):
    - → Males: 11 mg per day
    - → Females: 9 mg per day
- → Adults (19 years and older):
    - → Males: 11 mg per day
    - → Females: 8 mg per day

For pregnant and breastfeeding women,

- → Pregnant women: 11-12 mg per day, depending on age
- → Breastfeeding women: 12-13 mg per day, depending on age

(iii) What are the best vegetarian and non-vegetarian sources of zinc?

Vegetarian Sources:

→ Legumes: Lentils, chickpeas, kidney beans, black beans and other legumes

→ Seeds: Pumpkin seeds (pepitas), hemp seeds, flaxseeds, chia seeds and sesame seeds

→ Nuts: Cashews, almonds and pine nuts

→ Whole grains: Wheat germ, quinoa, oats and brown rice

→ Dairy products: Milk, cheese and yoghurt

Non-vegetarian sources:

Animal-based sources of zinc include:

→ Meat: Beef, pork and lamb

→ Seafood: Oysters are particularly high in zinc. Other seafood like crab, shrimp and lobster also provide zinc.

→ Poultry: Chicken and turkey

→ Eggs: Eggs, especially the yolks

→ Fish: Some types of fish, such as salmon and sardines

Biotin

If you want longer, healthier hair, then don't forget about biotin. Biotin, also known as vitamin B7 or vitamin H, is quickly becoming one of the most widely used supplements for faster hair growth. Biotin helps convert the nutrients from our diet into energy that supports hair follicle function and promotes hair growth.

While biotin is a B vitamin, it plays such a key role in keeping hair healthy that it earned its own spot on this list. This vitamin helps convert carbohydrates into glucose and activates amino acid metabolism in the fingernails and hair root cells. Since hair itself contains keratin, which is a form of protein, this supports healthy locks. While most people get enough biotin from the foods they eat each day, it is a water-soluble vitamin. Again, that means your body can't retain it and flushes what it doesn't use. So you need to get enough of it each day, or you'll run short.

(i) What does low biotin intake lead to?

Low levels of biotin in the body can lead to hair problems such as thinning, brittleness and slow hair growth. Biotin deficiency is relatively rare but can occur in individuals with certain conditions like malabsorption disorders, long-term antibiotic use or prolonged consumption of raw egg whites (which contain a biotin-binding protein). Additionally, people with genetic disorders affecting biotin metabolism may also be at risk of deficiency.

(ii) What is the recommended dosage of biotin?

The recommended daily intake of biotin, also known as vitamin B7 or vitamin H, can vary depending on age, sex and life stage. The following are the general guidelines for daily biotin intake, expressed in micrograms (mcg):

For most people,

- → Infants (0–6 months): 5-6 mcg per day
- → Infants (7–12 months): 6–8 mcg per day
- → Children (1–3 years): 8–12 mcg per day
- → Children (4–8 years): 12–20 mcg per day
- → Children (9–13 years): 20–25 mcg per day
- → Adolescents (14–18 years): 25–35 mcg per day
- → Adults (19 years and older): 30 mcg per day

For pregnant and breastfeeding women,

- → Pregnant women: 30 mcg per day
- → Breastfeeding women: 35 mcg per day

(iii) What are the best vegetarian and non-vegetarian sources of biotin?

Vegetarian Sources:

- → Nuts and seeds: Almonds, walnuts, peanuts, flaxseeds and chia seeds
- → Legumes: Lentils, chickpeas and soybeans
- → Whole grains: Brown rice, oats and barley
- → Vegetables: Spinach, broccoli, sweet potatoes and cauliflower
- → Fruits: Bananas, avocados and berries

Non-vegetarian sources:

- → Organ meats: Liver and kidney
- → Eggs: Egg yolks are particularly rich in biotin.
- → Fish and seafood: Salmon, tuna, mackerel and oysters

Omega-3 Fatty Acids

As the hair shaft contains about 3 per cent omega-3 fatty acids, this particular fatty acid is essential for maintaining healthy hair. Essential fatty acids, particularly omega-3 fatty acids, play a crucial role in maintaining healthy hair. They are important for nourishing the scalp, promoting hair growth, preventing hair loss, and improving the overall quality and appearance of the hair.

Omega-3 fatty acids, such as EPA (eicosapentaenoic acid) and DHA (docosahexaenoic acid), are considered essential because our bodies cannot produce them on their own and they must be obtained through our diet. These fatty acids help to nourish the hair follicles, reduce inflammation in the scalp, and improve blood circulation, all of which contribute to healthier and stronger hair.

Omega-3s work their magic by reducing scalp inflammation, ensuring your hair follicles are in their happy place for optimal growth. Say goodbye to pesky hair thinning and shedding!

EPA (eicosapentaenoic acid) and DHA (docosahexaenoic acid) are two important omega-3 fatty acids that play specific roles in nutrition for hair health:

EPA: EPA has anti-inflammatory properties, which can help reduce inflammation in the scalp. Inflammation can disrupt hair growth and contribute to hair loss. By reducing inflammation, EPA promotes a healthier scalp environment for hair follicles to thrive. It also helps improve blood circulation in the scalp, ensuring that essential nutrients and oxygen reach the hair follicles and promoting their growth and vitality.

DHA: DHA is a structural component of the cell membranes in the scalp and hair follicles. It helps to maintain the integrity and strength of these cell membranes, which are essential for healthy hair growth. DHA also contributes to the overall health of the scalp by providing nourishment and support to the hair follicles.

Both EPA and DHA are involved in maintaining the moisture balance of the scalp and hair. They help to keep the scalp hydrated, preventing dryness and itchiness, which can lead to dandruff and other scalp issues. Well-hydrated hair is less prone to breakage and appears more lustrous and shiny.

Guess what? Omega-3s are not only hair superheroes, but they also play a crucial role in keeping your hair strands strong, flexible and resistant to breakage. No more battles with brittle ends or split hair drama!

(i) What does low omega-3 intake lead to?

Low omega-3 intake can lead to heart health issues, including increased risk of heart disease, elevated blood pressure, and inflammation. It may also affect brain function, contributing to cognitive decline, memory problems, and mood disorders like depression and anxiety.

Inadequate omega-3s can impact eye health, immune function, and skin and hair health, leading to dry skin and brittle hair. Omega-3s' anti-inflammatory properties are crucial for joint health, and low intake may worsen joint inflammation and discomfort. During pregnancy, omega-3s are vital for foetal development, and its deficiency may affect the baby's brain and eye development.

(ii) What is the recommended dosage of omega-3?

For most people,

→ EPA and DHA combined: At least 250–500 mg per day for healthy adults

For pregnant and breastfeeding women,

→ DHA: 300 mg per day during pregnancy and lactation

For children and adolescents,

→ DHA: 100–250 mg per day

For individuals with heart disease or high triglyceride levels,

→ Higher doses ranging from 1 to 4 grams per day may be recommended under professional guidance.

What are the best vegetarian and non-vegetarian sources of omega-3?

Vegetarian Sources:

→ Flaxseeds (and flaxseed oil): Flaxseeds are rich in alpha-linolenic acid (ALA), a plant-based omega-3 fatty acid.

- Chia seeds: Chia seeds are another excellent source of ALA, providing a good amount of omega-3s.
- Walnuts: Walnuts contain ALA and are a convenient and tasty way to add omega-3s to the diet.
- Hemp seeds: Hemp seeds are a source of ALA and other essential nutrients.
- Seaweed and algae: Some types of seaweed and algae, like spirulina and chlorella, provide a form of omega-3 known as DHA (docosahexaenoic acid).

Non-vegetarian Sources:

Fatty fish are abundant in EPA (eicosapentaenoic acid) and DHA. Some examples include

- Salmon
- Mackerel
- Sardines
- Trout
- Herring
- Fish oil supplements derived from fatty fish are a concentrated source of EPA and DHA.
- Krill oil is extracted from tiny shrimp-like crustaceans called krill and contains both EPA and DHA.
- Fish roe, such as caviar, is a source of omega-3s.
- Cod liver oil is a supplement derived from the liver of codfish, providing EPA, DHA and vitamin D.

Selenium

Selenium is an essential trace mineral that plays a crucial role in maintaining healthy hair. It is a key component of enzymes called selenoproteins, which have antioxidant properties and help protect cells from damage. Selenium is involved in the production of glutathione peroxidase, an antioxidant enzyme that helps neutralize free radicals. This protects the hair follicles and scalp from oxidative stress, which can contribute to hair damage and hair loss. Selenium is required for the conversion of thyroid hormones from their inactive to active forms, as proper thyroid function is essential for healthy hair growth and maintenance.

(i) What does low selenium intake lead to?

Low selenium levels can lead to weakened immune system function, making the body more vulnerable to infections. It may also contribute to thyroid problems, such as hypothyroidism, as selenium is involved in the production and metabolism of thyroid hormones. Additionally, selenium's antioxidant properties play a role in protecting cells from oxidative stress, which can impact cardiovascular health. Selenium deficiency may contribute to hair loss or thinning by disrupting normal hair follicle function. Inadequate selenium levels can result in dry, brittle hair that is prone to breakage. Selenium deficiency may cause changes in hair texture, making it dull and lifeless.

(ii) What is the recommended dosage of selenium?

The recommended daily intake of selenium can vary depending on age, sex and life stage.

The following are the general guidelines for daily selenium intake, expressed in micrograms (mcg):

For most people,

- Infants (0–6 months): 15 mcg per day
- Infants (7–12 months): 20 mcg per day
- Children (1–3 years): 20 mcg per day
- Children (4–8 years): 30 mcg per day
- Children (9–13 years): 40 mcg per day
- Adolescents (14–18 years): 55 mcg per day
- Adults (19 years and older): 55 mcg per day

For pregnant and breastfeeding women,

- Pregnant women: 60 mcg per day
- Breastfeeding women: 70 mcg per day

(iii) What are the best vegetarian and non-vegetarian sources of selenium?

Vegetarian Sources:

- Brazil nuts
- Legumes: Beans, lentils and chickpeas
- Whole grains: Brown rice, quinoa, oats and wheat germ
- Seeds: Sunflower seeds and chia seeds
- Mushrooms: Some varieties of mushrooms, such as shiitake and white button mushrooms

Non-vegetarian Sources:

Seafood: Fish and shellfish are excellent sources of selenium. Some examples include:

- → Tuna
- → Salmon
- → Shrimp
- → Sardines
- → Cod
- → Crab
- → Meat: Poultry, beef and pork
- → Eggs: Eggs, especially the yolks

Silica

Silica, also known as silicon dioxide, is a trace mineral that plays a vital role in promoting healthy hair growth and maintaining the overall quality of our hair. It is a key component of the hair structure, contributing to its strength, elasticity, and shine. Silica helps in the formation of collagen, a protein that provides structure and strength to our hair strands. It improves hair elasticity, making it less prone to breakage and damage. Silica supports the growth of hair follicles by nourishing the scalp and promoting blood circulation. Adequate silica levels can help stimulate hair follicles, leading to healthier and faster hair growth. Silica has a soothing effect on the scalp and can help alleviate scalp conditions like dryness, itching, and dandruff. A healthy scalp is essential for promoting optimal hair growth.

(i) What does low silica intake lead to?

Low levels of silica in the body can lead to various hair problems, including brittle hair, thinning, and slow hair growth. Insufficient silica intake can weaken the hair shafts, making them more susceptible to breakage. It can also contribute to dryness, dullness and lack of shine in the hair.

(ii) What is the recommended dosage of silica?

The recommended daily intake of silica varies depending on factors such as age, gender and overall health. However, there is no specific recommended dietary allowance (RDA) for silica. Most studies suggest that an intake of 20–30 mg of silica per day is sufficient for adults to support hair health.

(iii) What are the best vegetarian and non-vegetarian sources of silica?

Vegetarian Sources:

- → Whole grains: Oats, brown rice, barley and wheat
- → Fruits: Apples, bananas, strawberries and grapes
- → Vegetables: Bell peppers, leafy greens, beets, asparagus and cucumbers
- → Horsetail herb: Horsetail (Equisetum) is a plant known for its high silica content and is sometimes used in herbal preparations.
- → Mineral water: Some types of mineral water may naturally contain trace amounts of silica.

Non-vegetarian Sources:

- → Seafood: Salmon and mackerel, as well as shellfish like shrimp and oysters.

Water

Water is an essential component for maintaining healthy hair. It plays a vital role in keeping the hair shaft hydrated, promoting elasticity, and preventing dryness and brittleness. Adequate water intake is crucial for maintaining optimal hair health and preventing various hair-related issues. To maintain proper hydration for your hair, it is important to drink water throughout the day and not rely solely on beverages that may contain other ingredients or additives.

Incorporating water-rich foods into your diet, along with a balanced intake of fruits, vegetables and fluids, will help ensure optimal hydration for both your body and your hair.

(i) What does low water intake lead to?

Insufficient water intake can have negative effects on hair quality. When the body is dehydrated, it prioritizes other essential functions over hair health. This can lead to dry and brittle hair, scalp dryness and increased hair breakage. Inadequate hydration can also disrupt the natural moisture balance of the scalp, leading to scalp issues such as dandruff or itchiness.

(ii) What is the recommended dosage of water?

The recommended daily intake of water is as follows:

For most people,

→ About 3.7 litres (or about 15.5 cups) per day for men

→ About 2.7 litres (or about 11.5 cups) per day for women

(iii) What are the best vegetarian and non-vegetarian sources of water?

→ Fruits and vegetables: Cucumber, watermelon, oranges, strawberries and celery

→ Beverages: Fluids like herbal teas, unsweetened fruit juices and milk (non-dairy or dairy)

→ Soups and broths: Soups and broths made from water and vegetables

Summary

In this chapter, an in-depth exploration of the 13 essential nutrients crucial for hair health is presented, delving into their roles and importance in maintaining vibrant and strong hair. Each nutrient's specific functions, sources, and potential impacts on hair growth and quality are meticulously examined, providing readers with a comprehensive understanding of the intricate relationship between nutrition and hair health. Through detailed discussions on key vitamins, minerals, and other vital elements, this chapter offers valuable insights into optimizing dietary intake to promote optimal hair condition and vitality.

CHAPTER 9

CRUCIAL FOODS FOR HEALTHY HAIR

List of Top Foods Important for Hair Growth

The power of eating clean is vast. Besides offering you a healthy body and glowing skin, it aids in strengthening your hair follicles. This means that the dream volume and lustre you've always wanted for your hair are achievable through food. A balanced diet is the most important thing when it comes to healthy and beautiful hair. If you're someone who sincerely follows the best haircare regimen but is still experiencing hair loss, you have probably not been eating the right foods. So, get closer to your hair goals by reading about the foods packed with vitamins and minerals that should make it into your diet.

Here's a detailed explanation of each superfood for hair and how it contributes to hair health:

Spinach	Spinach is rich in iron, which helps carry oxygen to the hair follicles, promoting healthy hair growth. It is also packed with vitamins A and C, which aid in the production of sebum, a natural conditioner for the scalp.

Salmon	Salmon is an excellent source of omega-3 fatty acids, which nourish the hair follicles and promote a healthy scalp. It is also high in protein, which is essential for hair structure and growth. Additionally, salmon contains vitamin D, which contributes to hair follicle health.
Eggs	Eggs are a great source of protein, which is the building block of hair. They also contain biotin, a B vitamin that promotes hair growth and overall scalp health. Eggs are also rich in vitamins B12 and E, which help prevent hair loss.
Avocado	Avocado is a powerhouse of healthy fats, such as omega-3 fatty acids and monounsaturated fats. These fats help nourish and moisturize the scalp, promoting healthy hair growth. Avocado also contains vitamins E and C, which protect the hair from oxidative stress.
Sweet potatoes	Sweet potatoes are rich in beta-carotene, which the body converts into vitamin A. Vitamin A is important for the production of sebum, which keeps the scalp and hair moisturized. Sweet potatoes also contain vitamin C, which aids in collagen production for strong hair.

Greek yoghurt	Greek yoghurt is a protein-packed food that provides essential amino acids for hair growth. It also contains vitamin B5, which helps improve blood flow to the scalp, promoting hair growth. Greek yoghurt is also a good source of vitamin D, which contributes to hair follicle health.
Blueberries	Blueberries are rich in antioxidants, particularly vitamin C and vitamin E. These antioxidants protect the hair follicles from damage caused by free radicals. Blueberries also improve scalp circulation, promoting healthy hair growth.
Walnuts	Walnuts are a great source of omega-3 fatty acids, which nourish the hair follicles and promote hair growth. They also contain biotin, which strengthens hair strands and prevents breakage. Walnuts are also rich in vitamin E, which helps protect the hair from damage.
Lentils	Lentils are a plant-based protein source that provides essential amino acids for hair growth. They are also rich in iron, which helps carry oxygen to the hair follicles. Lentils contain zinc and biotin, which promote healthy hair growth and prevent hair loss.

Brazil nuts	Brazil nuts are a great source of selenium, a mineral that supports hair follicle health. Selenium helps prevent oxidative damage to the hair follicles and promotes healthy hair growth. It also contributes to scalp health and reduces dandruff.

AYURVEDIC HERBS FOR HAIR GROWTH: UNVEILING NATURE'S SECRETS

Ayurveda, an ancient system of medicine, offers a treasure trove of herbs that can promote healthy hair growth. These herbs have been used for centuries and are known for their natural properties that nourish the scalp, strengthen the hair follicles and stimulate hair growth. Let's explore the top five ayurvedic herbs that are renowned for their ability to support vibrant and lustrous hair.

- **Bhringraj** (*Eclipta alba*): Bhringraj is often referred to as the 'king of herbs for hair' in Ayurveda. It has been traditionally used to address hair loss, premature greying and scalp disorders. Bhringraj stimulates hair follicles, enhances blood circulation in the scalp, and promotes hair growth. It also helps reduce dandruff and dryness, making the hair healthier and shinier.

- **Amla** (*Emblica officinalis*): Amla, also known as Indian gooseberry, is a powerhouse of nutrients and antioxidants. It is rich in vitamin C, which helps in collagen synthesis and supports the overall health of hair follicles. Amla strengthens the hair shaft, prevents breakage and promotes hair growth. It also nourishes the scalp, reduces dandruff and adds shine to the hair.

- **Brahmi** (*Bacopa monnieri*): Brahmi is an herb known for its calming and rejuvenating properties. It helps reduce stress, a common factor contributing to hair loss. By calming the mind and balancing hormones, Brahmi indirectly supports healthy hair growth. It also strengthens hair roots, prevents hairfall and improves overall hair texture.

- **Neem** (*Azadirachta indica*): Neem is a powerful herb with antimicrobial and anti-inflammatory properties. It helps maintain a healthy scalp by combating scalp infections and dandruff. Neem also stimulates blood circulation, promoting hair growth. It can help with scalp conditions like itching, irritation and excess oiliness, ensuring a clean and nourished environment for healthy hair.

- **Hibiscus** (*Hibiscus rosa-sinensis*): Hibiscus is widely known for its ability to revitalize hair and promote hair growth. It strengthens hair follicles, prevents hairfall, and adds volume to the hair. Hibiscus also helps maintain the natural pH balance of the scalp and prevents dryness. Regular use of hibiscus can result in softer, shinier and more manageable hair.

Ayurvedic herbs can be used in various forms, including powders, oils and hair masks. You can prepare herbal hair oils by infusing these herbs in a carrier oil like coconut oil or sesame oil. Massage the oil into your scalp and leave it on for a few hours or overnight before washing it off. Herbal hair masks can be made by mixing powdered herbs with other ingredients like yoghurt, aloe vera or coconut milk and applying the mixture to the hair and scalp.

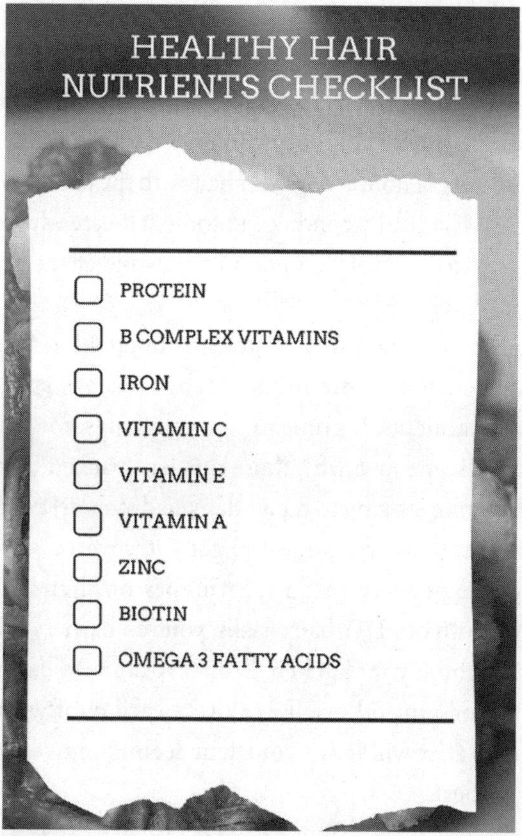

CHAPTER 10

HAIR MASKS

Welcome to the wonderful world of hair masks, where nutrition meets pampering for your locks! In this chapter, we'll dive deep into the secrets of nourishing your hair with the power of natural ingredients. Get ready to indulge in some self-care while treating your tresses to a feast of vitamins, minerals and all the good stuff your hair craves.

We all know that our hair goes through a lot, from daily exposure to environmental stressors to heat styling and chemical treatments. It's time to give your hair some extra TLC and show it some love with these nutrient-packed hair masks. Whether you're looking to repair damaged strands, boost shine, or add moisture to dry hair, we've got you covered.

Forget expensive salon treatments or chemical-laden products. With our DIY hair masks, you can harness the power of nature right in your kitchen. From avocados to bananas and honey to coconut oil, we'll explore a variety of wholesome ingredients that will leave your hair feeling rejuvenated and looking its best.

So, get ready to mix, blend, and apply these delicious concoctions to your hair. Sit back, relax, and let the nourishing goodness seep into every strand, providing your hair with the essential nutrients it needs to thrive. Get ready to unlock the secrets of healthy, vibrant hair with our hair masks that are as good for your hair as they are for your soul. It's time to take your haircare routine to the next level, one nourishing mask at a time.

Let's dive into this exciting chapter and discover the magic of hair masks that will leave you with gorgeous, luscious locks. Get ready to unleash the natural beauty of your hair and embrace the journey towards healthy, happy hair.

Here are our favourite hair masks; let's have a look:

1. Egg Mask

Ingredients:

- 2 eggs
- 2 tablespoon curd (Optional)

Steps:

- → Crack open two eggs into a bowl and whisk them until they are well mixed.
- → Apply the egg mixture thoroughly on your scalp and hair, gently massaging it in.
- → Allow the mask to settle on your hair for one hour.
- → Rinse off the mask using cold water.
- → Use a mild shampoo to remove any lingering egg smell.
- → Neutralize the smell of eggs by using curd.

2. Shikakai–Gram Flour Mask

Ingredients:

- Shikakai powder
- Besan (gram flour)
- Water

Steps:

→ Take equal quantities (according to your hair length) of shikakai powder and besan (gram flour) in a bowl.

→ Add water gradually to the mixture to form a fine paste.

→ Apply the mask generously to your scalp and hair, ensuring even coverage.

→ Leave the mask on for about an hour to allow the ingredients to work their magic.

→ After the designated time, rinse the mask thoroughly with water.

→ Enjoy the benefits of this protein-rich mask, especially if you have dry hair.

Experience the nourishing properties of this shikakai–gram flour mask, which combines the goodness of shikakai and gram flour to provide deep hydration and nourishment to your hair. Say goodbye to dryness and hello to healthier, more manageable locks with this easy-to-make homemade hair mask.

3.Banana–Coconut Milk Mask Mix

Ingredients:

- 1 ripe banana
- ½ cup coconut milk

Steps:

→ Start by mashing a ripe banana until it forms a smooth, pulpy paste.

→ Add half a cup of coconut milk to the mashed banana and mix well until you achieve a creamy consistency.

→ Apply the mask generously to your scalp and hair, making sure to cover all areas.

→ Leave the mask on for approximately 30 minutes to allow the nourishing ingredients to penetrate your hair.

→ Rinse off the mask thoroughly with cold water, ensuring that no residue is left behind.

Indulge in this rejuvenating banana-coconut milk mask to nourish your hair, leaving it feeling soft, silky, and full of vitality.

4. Egg–Yoghurt Mask Mix

Ingredients:

- Eggs
- Olive oil
- Apple cider vinegar

Steps:

- → Mix two eggs, half a cup of yoghurt, a half cup of olive oil, and a half cup of apple cider vinegar. Blend them well to form a creamy consistency.
- → Now, apply this pack across your scalp and wrap your hair with aluminium foil.
- → Leave it for about 30 minutes before rinsing it off with cold water.

5. Coconut Milk Mix Mask

Ingredients:

- Thick coconut milk

Steps:

- → Take a sufficient amount of thick coconut milk.
- → Apply the coconut milk generously to your hair, ensuring complete coverage from roots to tips.
- → Leave the coconut milk on your hair for two to three hours to allow it to deeply nourish and moisturize your strands.
- → Rinse your hair thoroughly with water to remove the coconut milk.
- → Enjoy the benefits of coconut milk, such as promoting hair growth, enhancing softness and silkiness, and preventing hair breakage.

Experience the magic of coconut milk as it works wonders for your hair, leaving it healthy, vibrant, and rejuvenated.

Embrace the power of natural remedies and unlock the secret to luscious, beautiful locks.

6. Fenugreek Seed Mix Mask

Ingredient:

- Fenugreek seeds

Steps:

→ Soak three or four spoons of fenugreek seeds in water or coconut milk for ten to twelve hours.

→ After soaking, make a fine paste of the fenugreek seeds.

→ Apply the paste to your scalp, ensuring even coverage.

→ Leave the mask on your hair for half an hour to allow it to work its magic.

→ Rinse off the mask thoroughly with water.

Experience the benefits of fenugreek seeds, as they not only add sheen to your hair but also help prevent hair loss. Try this easy DIY hair mask and unlock the natural goodness for healthier, more vibrant hair.

7. Indian Gooseberry (Amla) Mix Mask

Ingredients:

- Amla, lemon juice and curd

Steps:

→ Take a few spoons of amla (*Phyllanthus emblica*) powder, mix it with lemon juice or curd, and apply it as a thick paste to the scalp.

→ Wash off after an hour. This will stimulate hair growth and prevent dandruff. It also prevents white and grey hair.

8. Lemon Juice Mix Mask

Ingredients:

- 1 lemon
- 2 tablespoons lemon juice
- 4 tablespoons coconut oil

Steps:

→ Take a slice of lemon and gently massage your scalp in circular motions. This helps maintain the pH balance of your scalp and promotes a healthier environment for hair growth.

→ Mix two tablespoons of lemon juice with four tablespoons of coconut oil in a bowl. Stir well to ensure they are thoroughly combined.

→ Apply the lemon juice and coconut oil mixture to your scalp and hair. Massage it gently, focusing on the roots and ends. This nourishing blend helps improve hair growth and prevent split ends.

→ After applying the mask, leave it on for approximately three hours to allow the beneficial properties to penetrate deeply into your hair and scalp.

→ Once the treatment time is over, rinse off the mask with cold water. Cold water helps seal the hair cuticles, leaving your locks smooth and shiny.

Get ready to unveil your revitalized, beautiful hair with the power of this refreshing lemon juice hair mask. Enjoy the benefits of natural ingredients and embrace a healthier haircare routine.

9. Flax Seed Mix Mask

Ingredients:

- Flax seeds: 2–3 tablespoons
- Water (soak them properly)

Steps:

→ Soak the flax seeds in water for a week.

→ Apply the soaked flax seeds to your scalp.

→ Leave it on for half an hour.

→ Rinse off with lukewarm water.

Get ready to nourish your scalp and promote healthy hair growth with this simple and natural flax seed hair treatment.

10. Hibiscus Mix Mask

Ingredients:

- 1 hibiscus flower
- Handful of hibiscus leaves
- 2 tablespoons of olive oil
- 2 tablespoons of shikakai (*Acacia concinna*) powder

Steps:

→ Take a hibiscus flower and make a paste using a blender or mortar and pestle.

- → In a bowl, mix the hibiscus flower paste with two tablespoons of olive oil.
- → For the hibiscus leaf and shikakai mix, grind a handful of hibiscus leaves and two tablespoons of shikakai powder together until you get a fine powder.
- → To use as a natural shampoo, take a small amount (about one tablespoon) of the hibiscus leaf and shikakai mix and mix it with water to create a paste.
- → Apply the hibiscus flower and olive oil mixture to your hair, focusing on the roots and tips. Leave it on for about 30 minutes.
- → Rinse off the hibiscus flower and olive oil mixture thoroughly with water.
- → Use the hibiscus leaf and shikakai mix as a shampoo by applying it to your wet hair, massaging it into the scalp, and rinsing it off.
- → Repeat this hair mask and shampoo routine regularly to enjoy the benefits of hibiscus, including preventing premature ageing of the hair and promoting smooth and thick hair.

Experience the natural wonders of hibiscus and embrace the secret to youthful-looking hair. Get ready to nourish and protect your locks with this easy and effective homemade haircare routine.

11. Neem Paste Mix Mask

Ingredients:

- Handful of fresh neem leaves
- Water

Steps:

→ Rinse a handful of fresh neem leaves thoroughly.

→ Place the neem leaves in a blender or mortar and pestle.

→ Add a small amount of water to create a thick paste consistency.

→ Blend or grind the neem leaves until a smooth paste is formed.

→ Apply the neem paste directly to your scalp, focusing on areas affected by dandruff or lice.

→ Gently massage the paste into your scalp using circular motions.

→ Leave the neem paste on your scalp for 30 minutes to an hour.

→ Rinse off the paste with lukewarm water.

→ Shampoo and condition your hair as usual.

Say goodbye to dandruff and lice with the natural power of neem paste. This simple DIY remedy, made with fresh neem leaves and water, helps maintain a balanced scalp pH, preventing dandruff and promoting a healthy scalp environment. Give it a try and enjoy the benefits of neem for your haircare routine.

12. Aloe Vera Mask

It not only cleanses your face but also surprises you with its wonderful effects on your hair. Do you want to boost your hair growth? Massage with aloe vera gel, which adds sheen and stimulates hair growth.

Ingredients:

- Fresh aloe vera gel
- Optional: a few drops of essential oil for fragrance

Steps:

→ Extract fresh aloe vera gel from the plant by carefully peeling off the outer layer and scooping out the gel using a spoon.

→ Transfer the aloe vera gel into a bowl and blend it until smooth.

→ Optional: Add a few drops of your favourite essential oil to the mixture for a pleasant fragrance. (optional).

→ Apply the aloe vera gel evenly to your scalp and hair, gently massaging it in circular motions.

→ Leave the mask on for 30 minutes to an hour to allow the nourishing properties to penetrate your hair follicles.

→ Rinse off the mask thoroughly with lukewarm water, ensuring that no residue remains.

→ Follow up with your regular haircare routine.

Indulge in this rejuvenating aloe vera hair mask regularly to experience its remarkable effects on your hair growth and overall hair health. Get ready to embrace lustrous, beautiful hair with the power of nature's remedy.

13. Avocado Banana Mash Mask

Ingredients:

- 1 ripe avocado
- 1 ripe banana

Steps:

→ In a bowl, mash the ripe avocado until it forms a smooth paste.

→ Mash the ripe banana separately until it is free of any lumps.

→ Combine the mashed avocado and banana in a bowl and mix well until they are thoroughly blended.

→ Apply the mixture to your hair, starting from the roots and working your way down to the ends.

→ Leave the mask on for about an hour to allow the nutrients to penetrate your hair.

→ Rinse off the mask with lukewarm water, ensuring that all residue is removed.

→ Follow up with your regular shampoo and conditioner routine.

Indulge in this nourishing avocado-banana mash mask to promote hair growth and achieve soft, healthy-looking hair.

NOTE: Remember, the quantity of ingredients may vary based on your hair length. Adjust the quantities accordingly.

Congratulations! You've now unlocked the secret to luscious, healthy locks with fabulous hair masks. These natural wonders are packed with nutrient-rich ingredients that can transform your hair from dull to dazzling. Whether you're looking to boost hair growth, banish dryness or add that extra shine, these hair masks have got you covered.

Remember, the key to reaping the full benefits of these masks lies in consistency. Make them a regular part of your haircare routine, and your tresses will thank you. So, go ahead and treat yourself to some self-care sessions with these nourishing hair masks. Your hair will feel rejuvenated, and you'll rock those beautiful locks with confidence.

But wait, there's more! Our haircare journey doesn't end here. In the next chapter, we'll explore more tips and tricks for maintaining your hair's health and beauty. From styling secrets to expert advice, get ready to elevate your hair game to a whole new level!

Stay tuned for more exciting insights, and remember, the secret to fabulous hair begins with love, care, and these amazing hair masks!

Happy haircare!

Happy masking!

CHAPTER 11

HAIRCARE ROUTINE

Hey there, luscious locks enthusiasts! Get ready to dive into the wonderful world of haircare routines. We all know how much we adore our hair, and taking care of it should be a no-brainer, right? Well, in this chapter, we'll spill the beans on how the right tricks can work magic on your mane.

Additionally, we will share expert advice on proper cleansing and conditioning methods, choosing the right products for your hair type, and debunking common haircare myths. Get ready to embrace a holistic approach to haircare that not only addresses external factors but also nurtures your hair and scalp from the inside out.

So, whether you're a haircare enthusiast looking to refine your routine or someone seeking guidance to embark on a hair transformation journey, this chapter will provide you with the knowledge and inspiration to unlock the full potential of your tresses. Get ready to embrace a new level of self-care and discover the joy of beautiful, healthy hair. Let's begin this exciting chapter together!

Go, grab a cup, relax, and let's embark on this exciting journey to unlock the secrets of a fabulous haircare routine!

HAIRCARE ROUTINE FOR NORMAL HAIR

How you wash your hair and the products you use can go a long way towards maintaining smooth, shiny hair. Follow these simple tips to maintain healthy hair.

- ➢ **Wash oily hair more frequently:** How often you wash your hair should be based on how much oil your scalp produces.
  - If your scalp is oily, you may need to wash it as often as once a day.
  - If you have chemically treated hair, your hair may be drier, so you may want to wash it less frequently.
  - As you get older, your scalp makes less oil, so you may not need to shampoo as often. But if you see flakes in your hair, you may not be shampooing enough. This can lead to dandruff and other scalp diseases.
- ➢ **Concentrate shampoo on the scalp:** When washing your hair, concentrate on cleaning primarily the scalp rather than washing the entire length of hair. Washing only your hair can create flyaway hair that is dull and coarse.
- ➢ **Use conditioner after every shampoo:** Unless you use a 2-in-1 shampoo, which cleans and conditions hair. Using a conditioner can significantly improve the look of damaged or weathered hair by increasing shine,

decreasing static electricity, improving strength and offering some protection from harmful UV rays.

- **Concentrate conditioner on the tips of the hair:** Because conditioners can make fine hair look limp, they should only be used on the tips of the hair and not on the scalp or length of the hair.
- **Choose a shampoo and conditioner formulated specifically for your hair type:** For example, if you colour your hair, use a shampoo designed for colour-treated hair. If your hair is damaged or chemically treated, consider a 2-in-1 shampoo. Regardless of cost, many shampoo and conditioner brands provide the same benefits.
- **Protect hair when swimming:** Protect your hair from the damaging effects of chlorine by wetting and conditioning it before swimming. Wear a tight-fitting swim cap and use a specially formulated swimmer's shampoo and deep conditioner after swimming to replace lost moisture.

HAIRCARE ROUTINES FOR DIFFERENT HAIR CONDITIONS

Oily roots and dry ends hair

- → Washing hair with cold water; thus focusing on the scalp and lathering up only at the top.
- → Applying hydrating conditioner at the ends.
- → Air-drying hair or using heat tools can be used occasionally.

Greasy hair and a dandruff-prone scalp

- → Use anti-inflammatory agents like aloe vera and other mild shampoos to calm the scalp down, thus preventing flakes from forming.
- → Use a sulphate- and paraben-free anti-dandruff shampoo to cleanse the scalp, while conditioning only the very ends if need be.
- → Brushing the hair through is important, as this redistributes the oils from the top to bottom in a balanced manner.

Damaged lengths and oily roots hair condition

- → Choose keratin-building treatments and focus on strengthening the ends while deep-cleansing the scalp.
- → For best results, use a multi-mask with a clay-based scalp mask or an exfoliating scalp tonic/scrub while fortifying the ends and mid-lengths with a conditioning agent.

Checkout the harmful and safe chemicals in your hair products:

Chemicals harmful for your hair	• Formaldehyde • Isopropyl alcohol • Phthalates • Propylene glycol • Parabens • Silicones

	• Sulphates • Fragrances • Mineral oils and petroleum
Safe chemicals for your hair	• Sarcosines • Sulfosuccinates anionic detergents • Betaines • Sultaines • Imidazolinium derivatives • Sodium lauryl sulfoacetate (SLSA) • Sodium cocoyl glycinate • Sodium cocoyl glutamate • Disodium • Sodium lauroyl methyl isethionate • Sodium lauroyl taurate • Sodium lauroamphoacetate • Decyl glucoside • Lauryl glucoside

Many women use hair products every day to maintain the look they want for their hairstyle. Hair products can be detrimental to your hair if you choose the wrong type of product for your hair type and texture. Some common types of hair products include sulphates, parabens (USDA), polyethylene glycols, phthalates, formaldehyde, etc., which can be harmful to you. They most often leave your hair with a frizzy texture, and some even put you at risk for breast cancer. They also make your hair less wavy or curly by straightening or curling your strands.

Women with curly hair should stay away from these products since they can negatively affect the health of their curls by making them appear frizzy instead of bouncy and healthy-looking. Other negative effects of using these types of products include dandruff and dryness as well as split ends or brittle ends in your hair due to poor hygiene practices later in life.

CHAPTER 12

GUIDELINES FOR HEALTHY HAIR

1. Keep Protein Handy

Stock up on your protein-rich snacks!

Your hair is nearly 90 per cent protein, but as a non-essential function, hair growth is not a priority for your body. That's why, if you're interested in long, healthy and strong hair, protein needs to be a top priority in your diet. Protein is made up of amino acids. Your body needs twenty different amino acids to function properly. Nine of these amino acids are essential; we must consume them through our diet. This means that the key to protein intake is variety. Each protein source is made up of different amino acids in different amounts. I recommend keeping a variety of protein sources in your kitchen for optimal hair health.

2. Include Healthy Fats Daily

Dietary fats are an essential part of a healthy diet. They provide energy, increase vitamin uptake and support cell function.

Healthy fats like walnuts, avocado, extra-virgin olive oil and coconut oil nourish your hair follicles to give your hair strength and shine, and they can even reduce hair loss!

3. Eat Veggies and Fruits Regularly

Did you know that only 9 per cent of American adults consume the recommended amount of vegetables in their diet? This surprisingly low intake has significant nutritional consequences.

We know how important it is to have a variety of veggies and fruits in our diet for optimal health. Plants provide our body with vitamins, minerals, phytonutrients, polyphenols and phytochemicals, all of which play crucial roles in our health.

The next time you're grocery shopping, challenge yourself to get at least one plant from every colour of the rainbow.

4. Hydrate Adequately

Drinking enough water is essential to health and wellness! Proper hydration allows every system in the body to function properly, and because we are made up of about 60 per cent water, it's best to sip generously. From skin to scalp, water offers us an easy and natural way to support our hair's wellness, especially when it comes to growing hair, keeping the scalp healthy and maintaining a beautiful texture. Drinking enough water helps energize and support hair growth from root to tip. It also helps prevent split ends and a brittle hair texture, as well as foster a healthier scalp, meaning you'll have fewer chances of developing problems like dryness, itchiness, or dandruff. So how much water should you be sipping? A great starting point is to eat half of your body weight in ounces daily. This means if you weigh 120 lbs, you should be aiming for at least 60 oz of water each day.

5. Strive for Blood Sugar Balance

Unless you have a form of diabetes, you don't tend to think about your blood sugar very often. However, from a nutrition and hair wellness perspective, it may be a good time to start! When we eat a meal, our blood glucose will initially rise, and then our body will use insulin to lower those glucose levels to a normal range. This rise and fall should take a few hours if your blood sugar is well balanced. For some, this fall can be rapid (a crash) and leave you feeling hungry, cranky and low on energy. Internally, a dramatic blood sugar fall can also create stress in your body, which can lead to telogen effluvium. In telogen effluvium, significant stress pushes large numbers of hair follicles into a resting phase. Within a few months, affected hairs might fall out suddenly when simply combing or washing your hair. But don't fret too much; the good news is that telogen effluvium is completely reversible! So what should you eat to help balance your blood sugar? It's quite simple: Have fibre, fat and protein each time you eat! Fibre, fat and protein all help to slow down digestion, promoting a slower rise and fall of blood glucose.

6. Practise Mindful Eating

Just like blood sugar imbalances can cause stress in the body, the stressors around us (like work deadlines or relationship stressors) can wreak havoc on our digestion and our overall health. This is where mindful eating can be so impactful! Mindful eating is an eating practice based on Buddhist mindfulness principles. It uses mindfulness to reach a state of full attention to your experiences, cravings and physical cues when eating and supports more efficient digestion. To practise mindful eating, it's important to focus on your meal with as few distractions as possible—so no TV during dinner time! Here's what else you should do:

- Focus your attention on the flavours and textures of each bite.
- Eat slowly and chew thoroughly.
- Tune into how your food is making you feel.
- Stop eating when you feel naturally full.
- Enjoy the meal!

NUTRITION GUIDELINES FOR HEALTHY HAIR

Here are some nutrition and lifestyle guidelines for healthy hair, along with the dos and don'ts:

- **Eat a balanced diet:** Consume a nutrient-rich diet that includes a variety of fruits, vegetables, whole grains, lean proteins, and healthy fats. These provide essential vitamins, minerals, and antioxidants necessary for healthy hair growth.

- **Get sufficient protein:** Protein is the building block of hair, so ensure an adequate intake of high-quality proteins like lean meats, poultry, fish, eggs, legumes, nuts, and seeds.

- **Include healthy fats:** Healthy fats, such as omega-3 fatty acids found in fatty fish, flaxseeds, and chia seeds, are important for scalp health and hair moisture.
- **Stay hydrated:** Drink plenty of water to maintain hydration, as dehydration can lead to dry and brittle hair.
- **Consume nutrient-rich foods:** Incorporate foods rich in specific hair-nourishing nutrients such as iron (leafy greens, legumes), biotin (eggs, nuts, seeds), vitamin E (spinach, almonds), and vitamin C (citrus fruits, berries) into your diet.

LIFESTYLE GUIDELINES FOR HEALTHY HAIR

- **Practise good hair hygiene:** Wash your hair regularly with a mild shampoo and conditioner to keep the scalp clean and free from excess oil, dirt, and product buildup.
- **Avoid overwashing and harsh treatments:** Overwashing can strip the natural oils from the hair, leading to dryness. Also, minimize the use of harsh treatments like chemical relaxers, perms, and excessive heat styling.
- **Protect from heat and UV damage:** Use heat-protective products and avoid excessive use of hot styling tools. Additionally, shield your hair from UV damage by wearing a hat or using hair products with UV protection.

- **Manage stress:** Chronic stress can contribute to hair loss and affect hair health. Practise stress-management techniques like meditation, yoga, deep breathing exercises or engaging in activities you enjoy.

- **Avoid excessive manipulation:** Limit the use of tight hairstyles, excessive brushing, and harsh hair accessories that can cause hair breakage or traction alopecia.

- **Brush your hair before you shower:** No matter what your hair texture is, taking sixty seconds to detangle strands will keep them strong. When your hair is wet, it is more vulnerable to breakage, so always brush knots out of your hair when it's dry.One added benefit: brushing dry hair distributes the natural oils from your scalp down to the ends of your hair. Another plus: post-shower, it's already smooth and ready to style!

- **Condition correctly and with care:** Unless your hair is long, a nickel-size drop of conditioner is plenty for most textures and lengths. Apply your conditioner first to the mid-shaft and ends of your hair, then work your way up to the scalp. It's important to make sure your scalp gets hydration as well. Leave it on for a full minute before washing it out.

- **Take time for hair masks:** To keep strands hydrated and smooth, use a moisturizing hair mask or deep conditioner at least once a week, and more frequently if you use hot tools regularly.

- **Be mindful of key ingredients:** Staring down the haircare aisle can be overwhelming. With endless haircare options, how do you choose one? As you pick out your products, narrow down your options by looking for strengthening ingredients that will nourish your strands.

- **Eat a balanced diet:** You already know that you are what you eat. Your hair is mostly made up of protein, so eating a balanced diet of protein-rich foods is important. Add these items to your grocery list:

  - Fish
  - Meat
  - Eggs
  - Beans

  Other good sources of hair food are berries, spinach, and avocados, along with anything else rich in vitamins C and E, which will help boost collagen production, resulting in stronger strands.

- **Take a deep breath:** Breathe in through your nose and out through your mouth. The little things make a big difference. Our body's stress can show in our hair and skin. According to Staufenbiel et al. (2013), studies found higher hair cortisol levels in many situations like athletes, shift work, and major life events. For mental health, depression usually shows higher cortisol in hair, while bipolar disorder only in late-onset cases. Anxiety might lead to lower cortisol levels. Remember, taking care of yourself is important for your body and mind. Now, keep calm and read on.

- **Turn down the temperature of your shower:** As soothing as a steamy shower may feel, taking a super hot shower on a daily basis can irritate your scalp and possibly weaken your hair as it grows out. Keep the temperature on the warm side, and at the end of the shower, do a quick cold-water rinse to seal the cuticles shut, boost shine, and maintain healthy hair.

- **Shield strands from the sun:** UV rays don't only cause damage to your skin, and the same goes for pollution. When you style your hair, apply a leave-in styler to protect your strands.

- **Don't skip your scalp:** Healthy hair starts with a healthy scalp. If you notice dryness, itching, or any scalp issues, your hair will be affected by this. To maintain a balanced scalp, go for clarifying the scalp with proper hair products, oils and hair washing routines.

- **Sleep on silk:** Make the most of your beauty sleep by swapping out your cotton pillowcase for a silk alternative. It protects the cuticle of your hair by reducing the amount of friction between your hair and the fabric. Another secret to reduce stress on strands: Sleep with your hair in a loose topknot—secured with a silk scrunchie—or try a low, loose braid if you have thick or textured hair to give you more control of your strands during the night.

- **Style smarter:** To minimize damage from heat styling, invest in professional hot tools that have ionic technology, which will infuse moisture into your hair as you style. Also, opt for a curling iron or straightener that is solid ceramic, rather than only having a ceramic coating: This will distribute heat evenly onto your hair, locking in your style quickly so you don't need to re-apply the iron continuously to get your desired look. Follow these smart steps when using hot tools:
    - Let your hair air-dry as much as possible before you blow-dry. If you have curly or wavy hair, pull it back into a tight bun on day one; then, the next day, use an iron to shape it.
    - Switch up your hot tool usage: After you shampoo, blow dry your hair; on day two, use a curling iron or straightener; on day three, slick strands back to avoid heat styling. Then wash and repeat.

- **Get a trim:** You need regular haircuts to ensure that your strands stay healthy and don't break off at the ends. If you don't want to lose a lot of length, ask your stylist for a 'dusting', so only the tips are snipped, which gets rid of damaged ends but maintains the length. It's recommended to go every two months, and if you have a short or defined cut, you will likely need to go sooner.

Dos for Healthy Hair

- Maintain a balanced and nutritious diet
- Protect your hair from excessive heat and UV damage
- Practise good hair hygiene and use gentle haircare products
- Manage stress levels through relaxation techniques
- Get regular trims to prevent split ends

Don'ts for Healthy Hair

- Follow crash diets or restrictive eating patterns that may lead to nutrient deficiencies
- Use harsh chemical treatments or excessive heat styling
- Over wash or excessively manipulate your hair
- Ignore scalp health or neglect regular haircare routines
- Ignore signs of hair damage or excessive hair loss

HANDY SNACKS:

Find below some of the handy snacks which promotes healthy hair. You can check out our "Nutracy Lifestyle" App for knowing the below snacks recipes.

- Nutracy lifestyle Beauty Collagen +
- A bowl of roasted chana +
- A bowl of Mix seeds and nuts +
- Healthy Snicker Bites +
- Amaranth almond laddo +

CHAPTER 13

HEALTHY HAIR HABITS

HAIR MYTHS DEBUNKED

Haircare is a topic that is often surrounded by numerous myths and misconceptions. These myths, passed down through generations, can lead to confusion about the best ways to care for our hair. In this guide, we will debunk some of the most common hair myths and provide evidence-based information to help you make informed decisions about your haircare routine.

Myth: Cutting your hair frequently makes it grow faster.

Fact: Cutting your hair does not affect its growth rate. Hair growth occurs at the roots, and trimming the ends has no impact on the speed of hair growth. However, regular trims can prevent split ends, which can make your hair look healthier and promote overall hair health.

Myth: Brushing your hair 100 strokes a day makes it shinier.

Fact: Excessive brushing can actually cause damage to your hair. Brushing too much can lead to hair breakage and can strip away natural oils, leaving your hair dry and dull. Instead, opt for gentle brushing when necessary and use a wide-toothed comb to detangle your hair.

Myth: Washing your hair every day is necessary to keep it clean.

Fact: Washing your hair daily can strip away its natural oils and may lead to dryness and scalp irritation. How often you should wash your hair depends on your hair type and lifestyle. For most people, washing every 2-3 days is sufficient to keep the hair clean and healthy.

Myth: Using hot oil treatments can repair damaged hair.

Fact: While hot oil treatments can add temporary moisture to the hair, they cannot repair damaged hair permanently. Damaged hair needs proper care and nourishment, which includes using protein-rich products and avoiding excessive heat styling.

Myth: Split ends can be repaired with hair products.

Fact: Once the hair strand is split, it cannot be repaired. Hair products can temporarily mask the appearance of split ends, but the only way to get rid of them is to trim the damaged ends regularly.

Myth: Plucking one gray hair will cause more to grow in its place.

Fact: Plucking gray hair will not cause more gray hair to grow. However, it is not recommended to pluck hairs, as it can damage the hair follicle and lead to hair thinning.

Myth: The more you shampoo, the cleaner your hair will be.

Fact: Overshampooing can strip away the natural oils from your scalp, leading to dryness and scalp issues. It's best to find a shampoo that suits your hair type and wash your hair as needed.

Myth: Tying your hair tightly will make it grow faster.

Fact: Hair growth is determined by genetics and overall health, not by how you style your hair. Tying your hair too tightly can actually cause damage to the hair follicles and lead to hair loss.

By debunking these common hair myths, we hope to empower you to make informed choices about your haircare routine. Remember that each person's hair is unique, and what works for one may not work for another. It's essential to listen to your hair's needs and choose products and practices that promote its health and vitality.

SEASONAL HAIRCARE

It involves adjusting your haircare routine and practices according to the changing seasons and the environmental conditions that come with them. Each season presents unique challenges and impacts on your hair, and tailoring your haircare approach accordingly can help maintain healthy, vibrant locks throughout the year. Let's explore the key aspects of seasonal haircare with nutrition and how you can take care of your hair during different seasons:

1. Spring Season

Haircare:

- → Conditioning: After the dry winter months, focus on deep conditioning treatments to restore moisture and nourishment to your hair.
- → Protection: As the weather warms up, protect your hair from sun exposure by wearing hats or using hair products with UV protection.
- → Trimming: Get a trim to remove any split ends that may have occurred during the winter, promoting healthy hair growth.

Nutrition:

- → Focus on consuming foods rich in vitamins A, C and E to promote hair growth and scalp health.
- → Increase your intake of fresh fruits and vegetables like spinach, carrots, and citrus fruits.
- → Hydrate well to combat dryness and keep your hair and scalp moisturized.

2. Summer Season

Haircare:

- → Hydration: Drink plenty of water to keep your hair and scalp hydrated, especially in hot and humid conditions.
- → Moisturizing: Use leave-in conditioners or hair oils to combat dryness caused by sun and chlorine exposure.
- → Limit heat styling: Minimize the use of hot styling tools to prevent further damage to your hair, as the sun's rays can already be quite harsh.

Nutrition:

- → Stay hydrated to counter the effects of hot weather and sun exposure on hair and scalp.
- → Consume foods high in antioxidants to protect hair from damage caused by UV rays.
- → Include omega-3 fatty acids in your diet to maintain hair strength and reduce inflammation.

3. Monsoon Season

Haircare:

- → Anti-frizz products: Invest in anti-frizz hair products to combat the humidity and frizziness caused by the rain.
- → Scalp care: Keep your scalp clean and dry to prevent fungal infections that can occur in humid conditions.
- → Detangling: Be gentle with your hair to avoid breakage, as wet hair is more prone to damage.

Nutrition:

- → Incorporate foods rich in zinc and selenium to combat scalp infections and dandruff.
- → Boost iron intake to prevent hairfall and maintain healthy hair growth.
- → Avoid excessive consumption of sugary and processed foods that can worsen scalp conditions.

4. Autumn Season

Haircare:

→ Nutrition: Consume a diet rich in vitamins and minerals to support hair health during the transition from summer to winter.

→ Protective styles: Consider protective hairstyles like braids or buns to shield your hair from colder, drier air.

Nutrition:

→ Prioritize foods containing biotin to support hair growth and maintain hair strength.

→ Include proteins like lean meats, eggs and legumes to prevent hair breakage and promote thickness.

→ Stay hydrated and consume foods high in antioxidants to counter oxidative stress on hair.

5. Winter Season

Haircare:

→ Hydrating shampoos: Use moisturising shampoos and conditioners to combat the dryness caused by indoor heating and cold weather.

→ Avoid wet hair: Refrain from going out with wet hair in freezing temperatures to prevent breakage due to the cold.

Nutrition:

→ Increase intake of vitamin D, as sunlight exposure is reduced during winter months.

- → Consume foods high in zinc and fatty acids to combat dryness and maintain hair's moisture.
- → Consider using natural oils like coconut or olive oil as a pre-shampoo treatment to nourish dry hair.

Year Round

Haircare:

- → Regular trims: Schedule regular trims to maintain healthy hair and prevent split ends from traveling up the hair shaft.
- → Balanced diet: Ensure you have a well-balanced diet with sufficient protein, vitamins, and minerals for strong, shiny hair.
- → Minimal heat styling: Limit the use of heat styling tools and always use a heat protectant when styling.

Nutrition:

- → Stay well-hydrated throughout the year to support overall hair health.
- → Eat a balanced diet with a variety of nutrients, including proteins, vitamins, and minerals.
- → Avoid crash diets or extreme restrictions, as they can lead to nutrient deficiencies that affect hair quality.
- → Minimize processed and sugary foods that can contribute to inflammation and affect scalp health.
- → Remember, your hair's needs can vary from season to season, and it's essential to be attentive to the changes

and adapt your haircare routine accordingly. By being mindful of seasonal factors and following these tips, you can keep your hair looking its best all year round.

ESSENTIAL OILS

Essential oils have gained popularity for their potential benefits in promoting hair health. Here are commonly used essential oils and their potential effects on hair growth and scalp conditions:

1. **Lavender Oil:** Lavender oil is known for its soothing and calming properties. When applied to the scalp, it may help improve blood circulation and promote hair growth. It may also help balance oil production, making it suitable for both dry and oily scalps. Additionally, lavender oil has antimicrobial properties that can help combat scalp conditions like dandruff and itching.
2. **Rosemary Oil:** Rosemary oil is believed to stimulate hair follicles and promote hair growth. It may help increase blood circulation to the scalp, which can support the delivery of nutrients to the hair follicles. Rosemary oil is also known for its antioxidant properties, which can help protect the scalp and hair from free radicals that may cause damage. It is often used to improve the overall health and appearance of the hair.
3. **Tea Tree Oil:** Tea tree oil is known for its antimicrobial and anti-inflammatory properties. It can help manage scalp conditions like dandruff, scalp itchiness, and scalp acne. Tea tree oil may help cleanse the scalp by removing

impurities and excess oil, which can contribute to a healthier scalp environment. However, it is important to use tea tree oil in diluted form to avoid potential skin irritation.

4. **Peppermint Essential Oil:** Peppermint oil is known for its refreshing and cooling properties. It helps to improve blood circulation to the scalp, which can stimulate hair follicles and promote hair growth. The menthol in peppermint oil has a soothing effect on the scalp and can help alleviate itchiness and irritation. Its antimicrobial properties also make it beneficial for maintaining a clean and healthy scalp.
5. **Cedarwood Essential Oil:** Cedarwood oil has been traditionally used to support hair growth and reduce hair loss. It helps balance oil production in the scalp, making it suitable for both dry and oily hair types. Cedarwood oil's antifungal properties can also help combat dandruff and other scalp issues. Its calming aroma makes it an excellent choice for aromatherapy to reduce stress, which can contribute to hair loss.
6. **Ylang-Ylang Essential Oil:** Ylang-ylang oil is known for its floral fragrance and its ability to promote hair thickness and growth. It helps balance the production of sebum in the scalp, which can lead to healthier hair and prevent excessive greasiness. Ylang-ylang oil's moisturizing properties can also improve the overall appearance and texture of the hair.

7. **Clary Sage Essential Oil:** Clary sage oil is another excellent option for promoting hair growth and reducing hair loss. It has natural astringent properties that can help regulate excess oil production in the scalp. This oil also contains linalyl acetate, which can soothe and calm the scalp, making it useful for those with an itchy or irritated scalp.
8. **Lemongrass Essential Oil:** Lemongrass oil has a refreshing citrusy scent and is beneficial for promoting a healthy scalp. It possesses antifungal and antibacterial properties that can help maintain scalp health and prevent dandruff and infections. Lemongrass oil's natural astringent properties can also help reduce excess oil and keep the scalp clean.

When using essential oils for haircare, it is important to dilute them with carrier oils like coconut oil, jojoba oil, or almond oil before applying them to the scalp. This helps prevent skin irritation and ensures safe usage. It is also recommended to perform a patch test before using any essential oil to check for any adverse reactions.

Remember, essential oils should not replace a comprehensive haircare routine or medical advice. If you have any specific scalp conditions or concerns, it is best to consult with a healthcare professional or a qualified aromatherapist for personalized guidance.

CHAPTER 14

RECIPES

SNACKS

1. Besan Methi Chilla

Ingredients	Method
• ½ cup besan • 2 tbsp methi leaves • ½ tsp salt • ½ turmeric powder • ½ hing • ½ coriander powder • ½ cup water	• Mix all the ingredients in a thin batter consistency. • Now pour scoops of this batter on a pan • Serve the chillas with green chutney and it's ready.

2. Cauliflower Green Salad

Ingredients	Method
• 1 medium cauliflower • ¼ cup curd • 1 tsp ginger-garlic paste • 1 tbsp besan • ¼ tsp turmeric powder • 1 tsp jeera • 1 tsp coriander powder • 1 tsp chilli powder • ½ tsp garam masala powder • 1 tsp kasuri methi • 1 tbsp ghee/oil • Salt as per taste	• Mix all the ingredients together, add steamed cauliflower florets. Let it marinate for at least an hour, and then grill it. • For salad, add cucumber, tomatoes, capsicum, pickled onions, ½ tsp red chilli flakes, salt in a bowl. Mix well. • Serve the cauliflower florets with salad and homemade green chutney!

3. Broccoli Tikkis

Ingredients	Method
• 1 cup broccoli florets • ¼ cup boiled potato • 1 tsp chopped ginger • 1 tsp chopped garlic • 1 green chilli • ¼ cup coriander leaves	• Mix broccoli with all the herbs and spices. • Next, make the mixture into tiny balls/cutlet shape. • Now, shallow fry these balls.

Ingredients	Method
• Salt to taste • ¼ tsp red chilli powder • ¼ tsp black pepper powder • ½ tsp coriander powder • ½ tsp cumin seeds • ½ tsp amchur/mango powder • ¼ tsp garam masala • 2 tbsp roasted gram flour • 1 tbsp roasted sesame seeds	• Serve the broccoli bites with green chutney and enjoy.

4. Fresh Fruit Bowl

Ingredients	Method
• ¼ cup green grapes • ¼ cup orange (peeled and chopped coarsely) • 1 ripe banana (peeled and sliced) • 2 tbsp fresh pomegranate fruit kernels • 1 kiwi (peeled and sliced) • 1 apple (chopped)	• Prepare all the chopped fruits first before starting to make the Fresh Fruit Bowl recipe. • After all the fruits have been cut and peeled (try using the peel of fruits that have an edible peel, such apples or chiku), place the fruits in a large

Ingredients	Method
• ¼ cup red grapes • Chaat masala powder (optional) • Salt and pepper (optional) • 1 tbsp lemon juice • 5 mint leaves	mixing utensil and gently toss to combine all the ingredients. • Serve the bowl of fresh fruits with mint leaves on top.

5. Smoky Sweetcorn Thick Tomato Soup

Ingredients	Method
• 600 ml vegetable stock • 75 g potato • 80 g sweetcorn • 3 gloves of garlic • 1 medium-sized onion (diced) • 1 medium tomato • 2 green chillies • 1 tsp turmeric powder • 2 tsp oil **To serve:** • 15 g chopped spring onion • 10 g chopped coriander	• Add the drained sweetcorn to a pot with 1 tsp oil and 2 tsp green chillies. • Stir over medium heat until the mixture is golden brown. • Next, add diced onion, tomato and garlic; stir until soft with 1 tsp oil. • Peel and chop the potatoes into 1-2 cm chunks. Add to the pot, and mix until everything is well coated.

Ingredients	Method
	• Pour in the stock and bring to a simmer. Let the soup simmer for 20 mins or until the stock has reduced slightly. • Remove ¼th of the potato and corn from the pot and keep it aside. • Add the rest of the soup to a blender and blend well until smooth. • Add the separated potato and corn back to the pot. • Stir well and season, along with serving ingredients, and enjoy.

MEAL

1. Golden Chickpea Salad

Ingredients	Method
• 1 cup chickpeas • 2 cups cooked quinoa • 1 tsp turmeric in the cooking water	• Finely chop all the vegetables in medium size. • Sauté all the base ingredients.

Ingredients	Method
• ½ cup tomato • 1 cup carrots • ⅓ cup onion • 1 cup steamed corn • 1 cup capsicum **Dressing** • 2 tbsp olive oil • ¼ cup peanut butter • 2 tbsp lemon juice • 1 tsp cumin • ½ tsp turmeric • 1 tsp salt • ¼ black pepper	• Place all the base ingredients in a large bowl. • Blend all the dressing ingredients in a small bowl first, and then pour this mix into the larger bowl of base ingredients. • Toss now all the ingredients. • Serve garnished with fresh coriander.

2. Sautéed Soya Chunks Curry

Ingredients	Method
• 75 g of soya chunks • 1 garlic clove, chopped • ½ cup onion, chopped • 1 tsp red chilli paste (soak dry chillies in water and grind to a smooth paste with a little water) • Tomato purée	• Add salt to soya chunks, immerse in hot water completely, and let the soya soften. • Drain the water completely. Add ½ tsp chilli powder, ¼ tsp turmeric powder, and salt. Pan-fry until golden.

Ingredients	Method
• ½ tsp salt • ½ tsp chilli powder • ¼ tsp turmeric powder • 1 tsp oil	• Then add 1 chopped garlic clove, ½ cup chopped onion, ¾ cup tomato purée, and 1 tsp red chilli paste. • Warm up 1 tsp oil. Sauté garlic, onions, tomato purée, and chilli paste mix. Cover and cook for 4–5 minutes until the raw smell leaves. • Add capsicum or any veggie, roasted soya, salt as required, and garam masala. Mix and sauté for a minute. • Switch off heat. Drizzle with lemon juice and coriander, and serve hot.

SMOOTHIES

1. Chocopro Smoothie

Ingredients	Method
• 1 tbsp unsweetened cocoa powder • 1 tbsp cacao nibs • 1 tbsp peanut butter • 1 scoop protein powder • 1 glass almond milk • ½ banana • 5 mint leaves • 1 tbsp chopped almonds	• Blend all the ingredients to a medium-thick consistency. Then add banana slices, mint leaves and 1 tbsp chopped almonds on top. Its ready!

2. Almond Coconut Butter Smoothie

Ingredients	Method
• ½ banana • 1 tbsp peanut butter • ¼ coconut milk • 1 tbsp chopped almonds • 2 tbsp sugar	• Blend all the ingredients to a thick consistency, and it's ready to consume.

3. Banana Mango Nuts Smoothie

Ingredients	Method
• Oats: 1 tbsp • 8 cashew nuts • 4 almonds • 3 walnuts • 1 tsp pumpkin seeds • 1 tsp muskmelon seeds • 1 medium size banana • ¼ cup mango • 1 cup water • ½ tsp chia seeds	• Soak all nuts and seeds in 1 cup of water overnight. • Blend all the ingredients and serve the smoothie in a glass.

4. Coconut Mango Mint Smoothie

Ingredients	Method
• ¼ cup soaked oats • ½ cup oats • ⅓ cup kiwi • 1 mango • 5 dates • ¼ cup fresh mint leaves • 2 tbsp overnight-soaked peanuts • 1 cup coconut milk • 2 tbsp soaked chia seeds	• Blend all the ingredients in a high-speed blender, and it's done.

CHAPTER 15

THE ACTION PLAN FOR GORGEOUS HAIR

This chapter outlines your plan of action for healthy and smooth hair. Check out the below-mentioned detailed steps that you can begin actioning upon today:

ACTION 1: AFFIRMATIONS

What are affirmations?

Affirmations for hair are positive statements or declarations that you repeat to yourself to create a positive mindset and belief system about your hair. They are intended to shift your thoughts and perceptions about your hair, promoting self-love, acceptance and appreciation for its natural state and beauty. Affirmations for your hair can help you develop a positive relationship with it, boost your confidence and foster a sense of gratitude and care for it. By repeating affirmations regularly, you reinforce positive beliefs and empower yourself to embrace and celebrate your hair, regardless of its texture, colour or style.

Why practise affirmations for hair health?

Practising affirmations for hair health can have several benefits:

- **Positive mindset:** Affirmations help cultivate a positive mindset and shift your focus from any negative thoughts or insecurities about your hair. By affirming positive statements about your hair, you can promote self-acceptance, love, and appreciation for your hair, enhancing your overall well-being.
- **Self-confidence:** Affirmations can boost your self-confidence and improve your self-image. When you repeat affirmations that emphasize the health and beauty of your hair, you begin to believe in your hair's natural qualities and feel more confident in your appearance.
- **Stress reduction:** Hair-related concerns can sometimes cause stress or anxiety. Affirmations for hair health can help alleviate these negative emotions by redirecting your attention to positive aspects of your hair and promoting a sense of calm and acceptance.
- **Haircare commitment:** Repeating affirmations for hair health can serve as a reminder and motivation to take good care of your hair. When you make positive statements about your hair, you are more likely to engage in healthy haircare practices, such as regular washing, conditioning, and protecting your hair from damage.
- **Mind–body connection:** Affirmations have the power to influence your mindset, emotions, and even your physical

well-being. By practising affirmations for hair health, you can foster a positive mind–body connection, which may contribute to improved hair health over time.

Remember that affirmations work best when combined with consistent actions and self-care practices. By affirming positive statements about your hair and supporting them with proper haircare routines, you can enhance your overall hair health and nurture a positive relationship with your hair.

How affirmations help with improving hair issues:

While affirmations alone may not directly address specific hair issues, they can contribute to an improved mindset and overall well-being, which can indirectly support hair health. Here's how affirmations can help with improving hair issues:

- **Confidence to tackle hair issues:** Affirmations boost your self-confidence and self-image. When you have a positive mindset and believe in the beauty and health of your hair, you may feel more confident in managing any hair issues.
- **Less stress make for happy hair:** Hair issues can often cause stress or anxiety. Practising affirmations can help reduce stress levels and promote a sense of calm. By managing stress, you create a more favourable environment for healthy hair growth and maintenance.
- **Helps prioritize haircare:** Affirmations can serve as a reminder to prioritize self-care, including haircare. By affirming positive statements about your hair, you

reinforce the importance of nurturing your hair through proper care practices, such as gentle handling, nourishing treatments and regular maintenance.

- **Overall wellbeing:** Affirmations foster a positive mindset and can help shift your focus away from perceived hair issues or shortcomings. By focusing on positive aspects of your hair, you cultivate a mindset that supports your overall well-being and may contribute to improved hair health over time.
- **Enhances patience and persistence:** Some hair issues require time and consistency to address effectively. Affirmations can help cultivate patience and persistence in your haircare journey. By affirming positive statements about your hair and its potential for improvement, you can stay motivated and committed to taking the necessary steps to address and improve hair issues.

Remember that affirmations work in conjunction with other practical measures to address specific hair issues.

The Science Behind It

While affirmations for improving hair issues may not have direct scientific evidence, they can contribute to psychological well-being, which indirectly impacts overall health, including hair health. Here are some aspects to consider:

- **Mind–body connection:** Research has shown that our thoughts and emotions can influence our physical health. Stress and negative emotions can impact our overall well-being, including our hair health. Affirmations help promote positive emotions, reduce stress, and foster a healthier mind–body connection, which can have a positive impact on hair health.

- **Self-perception and confidence:** Affirmations can influence self-perception and confidence. When you make positive statements about your hair, it can enhance your self-esteem, which may lead to better haircare practices and improved hair health.
- **Stress reduction:** Chronic stress has been associated with hair-related issues such as hair loss and thinning. By incorporating affirmations into your routine, you can promote relaxation, reduce stress levels and create a more favourable environment for healthy hair growth.
- **Motivation and consistency:** Affirmations can provide motivation and reinforce positive habits. When you affirm positive statements about your hair and haircare practices, it can encourage consistency in your routine, such as regular scalp massages, gentle handling, and using nourishing hair products, which can contribute to improved hair health over time.
- **Placebo effect:** Affirmations may also harness the placebo effect, where believing in the effectiveness of a treatment or practice can lead to actual physiological changes. When you genuinely believe in the power of affirmations for improving hair health, it can positively influence your mindset and potentially contribute to positive outcomes.

Remember, affirmations work best when integrated into your daily routine alongside proper haircare practices and seeking professional advice when needed.

Here are some affirmations you should practise in your daily routine. Take a break. Relax. Say these affirmations out loud, or you can write them down too.

#1 My hair is strong, vibrant, and full of life.

____

#2 I nourish my hair with love and care every day.

____

#3 I am grateful for my hair and appreciate its natural beauty.

____

#4 My hair grows abundantly and at a healthy pace.

____

#5 I embrace my unique hair texture and celebrate its beauty.

____

#6 I have a healthy scalp, and my hair follicles are thriving.

____

#7 I practise self-care rituals that promote the health and vitality of my hair.

____

#8 Each strand of my hair is filled with strength and resilience.

____

#9 I am patient and gentle when handling and styling my hair.

____

#10 I attract positive energy that supports the health and growth of my hair.

____

#11 I make choices that promote the longevity and radiance of my hair.

____

#12 My hair reflects my overall well-being, and I prioritize my health for healthy hair.

____

#13 I release any negative thoughts or beliefs about my hair and replace them with positivity and love.

____

#14 I give my hair the attention it deserves, using nourishing products and treatments.

____

#15 My hair is a reflection of my inner beauty and self-confidence.

____

Action 2: Exercises

Regular exercise offers several benefits that indirectly promote hair health:

- ☐ **Improved blood circulation:** Exercise increases blood flow throughout the body, including the scalp. This enhanced circulation delivers essential nutrients and oxygen to the hair follicles, supporting their growth and overall health.
- ☐ **Stress reduction:** Exercise is known to reduce stress levels by triggering the release of endorphins, the

feel-good hormones. Lowering stress levels is crucial for hair health, as high levels of stress can contribute to hair loss and other scalp-related issues.

- ☐ **Hormonal balance:** Engaging in physical activity helps maintain hormonal balance in the body. Hormonal imbalances, such as an excess of androgens (male hormones), can lead to hair thinning and loss. Regular exercise can help regulate hormone levels, promoting healthier hair growth.
- ☐ **Enhanced immune function:** Regular exercise strengthens the immune system, reducing the likelihood of scalp infections or conditions that could affect hair health. A robust immune system can help fight off infections that may hinder hair growth.
- ☐ **Increased nutrient absorption:** Exercise improves the body's ability to absorb and utilize nutrients from the diet. Proper nutrient absorption ensures that the hair follicles receive the necessary vitamins, minerals and proteins required for healthy hair growth.
- ☐ **Reduced DHT levels:** Dihydrotestosterone (DHT) is a hormone that can contribute to hair loss when present in excess. Exercise can help lower DHT levels by reducing the production and sensitivity to this hormone, promoting healthier hair growth.
- ☐ **Overall well-being:** Exercise contributes to overall well-being and a healthy lifestyle. When you take care of your body through regular physical activity, it positively impacts your hair and scalp health as well.

To promote hair health, you can incorporate the following exercises into your routine:

- ☐ **Scalp massage:** Gently massaging your scalp helps improve blood circulation, which promotes hair growth and nourishment. Use your fingertips to massage your scalp in circular motions for 5–10 minutes daily.
- ☐ **Yoga:** Certain yoga poses, such as the downward-facing dog or headstand, encourage blood flow to the scalp and reduce stress, which can benefit hair health. Practise yoga regularly to improve overall circulation and promote hair growth.
- ☐ **Cardiovascular exercises:** Engaging in cardiovascular exercises like jogging, cycling or swimming increases blood circulation throughout your body, including the scalp. This enhanced blood flow brings nutrients to the hair follicles, supporting healthy hair growth.
- ☐ **Headstands:** Inversion poses, like headstands, can improve blood flow to the scalp. Be cautious and ensure you have proper guidance and practise headstands safely to avoid any injuries.
- ☐ **Neck and shoulder stretches:** Tension and stress in the neck and shoulder region can affect hair health. Perform regular neck and shoulder stretches to relieve tension and improve blood circulation in the scalp.

- ☐ **Breathing exercises:** Deep breathing exercises, such as pranayama, help reduce stress levels, which can have a positive impact on your hair health. Practising deep breathing regularly can promote relaxation and provide optimal conditions for hair growth.
- ☐ **Resistance training:** Including resistance training exercises, like weightlifting or using resistance bands, in your workout routine can indirectly benefit hair health. Resistance training stimulates the release of growth factors and hormones that contribute to healthy hair growth.

Exercise 1: Scalp Massage

Scalp massages can indeed contribute to hair health in several ways. Here are some benefits of scalp massages and how they can promote healthier hair:

- ☐ **Increased blood circulation:** Massaging the scalp helps stimulate blood flow to the hair follicles, delivering essential nutrients and oxygen. Improved circulation nourishes the hair follicles, promoting healthier hair growth.
- ☐ **Stress reduction:** Scalp massages can be relaxing and help reduce stress and tension. Stress is known to contribute to hair loss and other hair-related issues. By reducing stress, you can minimize the negative impact it has on your hair.

- ☐ **Removal of buildup:** Massaging the scalp can help dislodge and remove product buildup, excess oil, and dead skin cells. This can improve the overall health of your scalp and hair, preventing issues like dandruff or scalp inflammation.
- ☐ **Stimulation of sebum production:** Gentle scalp massage can help stimulate the production of sebum, a natural oil produced by your scalp. Sebum acts as a natural conditioner, keeping your hair moisturized and protecting it from damage.
- ☐ **Relaxation and improved sleep:** Scalp massages can provide a sense of relaxation and tranquility, leading to improved sleep quality. Sufficient rest is crucial for overall health, including the health of your hair.

Tips for Scalp Massages:

- Use your fingertips or the pads of your fingers to massage your scalp in circular motions. Apply gentle pressure without causing discomfort.
- Consider using natural oils like coconut oil, olive oil, or jojoba oil for added benefits. Apply a small amount to your fingertips and massage it into your scalp.
- You can also use a scalp massager tool, such as a handheld massager with soft bristles or rounded tips, to enhance the massage experience.
- Practise regular scalp massages, ideally a few times a week, to enjoy the long-term benefits.

Exercise 2: Yoga

☐ **Downward-facing dog pose**

To practise the downward-facing dog pose, also known as Adho Mukha Svanasana in Sanskrit, follow these steps:

- Start on your hands and knees, aligning your wrists directly under your shoulders and your knees directly under your hips. Spread your fingers wide apart and press firmly into your palms.
- Curl your toes under and, on an exhale, lift your knees off the ground, straightening your legs. Your body will form an inverted V shape.
- Press your palms into the mat, lengthening your spine and engaging your core. Allow your head and neck to relax, allowing your gaze to fall between your legs or towards your belly button.
- Keep your heels slightly lifted off the ground and focus on lengthening your spine, reaching your tailbone up towards the ceiling.
- Press your thighs back and apart, engaging your quadriceps. Feel a gentle stretch in the back of your legs.
- Maintain an even weight distribution between your hands and feet. If needed, you can slightly bend your knees or adjust the position of your hands to find a comfortable position.

- Breathe deeply and hold the pose for several breaths, aiming to gradually increase your hold time as you become more comfortable.
- To release the pose, gently bend your knees and lower them back to the mat, returning to the starting position on your hands and knees.

Tips:

- If you're a beginner or have tight hamstrings, it's normal for your heels to be off the ground. Focus on the lengthening of your spine and the engagement of your core.
- Modify the pose as needed to ensure comfort and avoid strain or pain.
- As with any yoga pose, listen to your body and make adjustments accordingly. If you have any specific concerns or conditions, it's advisable to consult with a qualified yoga instructor.
- Practising downward-facing dog regularly can help improve flexibility, strengthen the upper body, stretch the back of the legs, and promote overall body awareness and relaxation.

☐ Headstand

Performing a headstand, also known as Sirsasana in yoga, requires strength, balance and proper technique. It is an advanced pose, so it's essential to approach it with caution and ensure you have developed the necessary strength and stability. Here's a general guide on how to practise a headstand:

- Find a clear, uncluttered space and place a folded yoga mat or blanket on the ground for cushioning.
- Start by kneeling on the mat with your forearms resting on the ground parallel to each other. Interlace your fingers, forming a stable base for your head. Your elbows should be shoulder-width apart.
- Place the top of your head against the mat with the back of your head cradled in your hands. The position of your hands and forearms should create a triangle with your head at the apex.
- Tuck your toes and straighten your legs, lifting your hips towards the ceiling. Walk your feet closer to your head, creating a stable foundation and preparing for the inversion.
- Engage your core muscles and press your forearms and hands firmly into the mat. Slowly lift your knees off the ground, shifting your weight onto your forearms and head.
- Gradually extend your legs upward, engaging your core and legs to maintain balance. Keep your gaze relaxed, focusing on a point between your hands or slightly in front of you.
- Find stability and balance in the pose, keeping your body aligned. Continue to engage your core, glutes, and leg muscles to maintain control.

- Breathe deeply and hold the pose for a desired duration, gradually increasing your practise time as you gain strength and confidence. To come out of the headstand, slowly lower your legs back down with control and return to a kneeling position.

Important Considerations:

- Practise headstands under the guidance of an experienced yoga instructor if you are a beginner or new to inversions.
- Ensure that you have no neck or head injuries, high blood pressure, or any conditions that contraindicate inversions.
- It's crucial to build strength and stability in your upper body, core, and shoulders before attempting headstands.
- Never force yourself into a headstand. Progress gradually, listening to your body, and respecting its limits.
- Seek professional guidance, practise with caution, and prioritize safety while learning and practising headstands or any advanced yoga pose.

Exercise 3: Resistance Training

Ready to take your fitness game to the next level? Incorporating resistance training exercises, like weightlifting or bodyweight exercises, into your routine is a game-changer for building muscle and improving your body composition. Guess what? Your skin will thank you too!

Resistance training is like giving your muscles a wakeup call. When you challenge your muscles by lifting weights or engaging in bodyweight exercises, you're stimulating muscle growth and increasing muscle tone. This not only helps you achieve that sculpted, toned look but also has a positive impact on your skin.

Exercise 4: Pilates

Pilates is all about strengthening your core, improving flexibility and developing body awareness. Through controlled movements and specific breathing techniques, Pilates engages multiple muscle groups. By practising Pilates, you can improve your posture, enhance circulation and achieve overall body tone, which can positively impact the appearance of your skin.

How can pilates help you

- **Enhanced Circulation**

  One of the significant benefits of Pilates is its ability to improve circulation throughout the body. The controlled movements and muscle engagement in Pilates encourage blood flow to all areas, including the skin. With improved circulation, the skin receives a greater supply of oxygen, essential nutrients and immune cells. This nourishment supports the skin's health and vitality, promoting a radiant complexion and aiding in the repair and rejuvenation of skin cells. The increased blood flow also aids in the removal of toxins and waste products from the skin, contributing to a clearer and more vibrant appearance.

- **Stress Reduction**

  Pilates is not just a physical exercise; it is a mind-body practice that emphasizes mindfulness and body awareness. Through focused breathing techniques and intentional movements, Pilates helps activate the body's relaxation response, reducing stress levels and promoting a sense of calm. Chronic stress can have detrimental effects on the skin, leading to inflammation, breakouts, and accelerated ageing. By engaging in Pilates, you can effectively manage stress, minimizing its negative impact on the skin. The release of tension and the promotion of relaxation through Pilates can help restore balance in the body, improving overall well-being and promoting a healthy complexion.

Are you ready to start your Pilates routine? Consider incorporating the following exercises into your practice:

- **The Hundred**

  Lie on your back with your knees bent and lift your head and shoulders off the mat. Extend your legs to a 45-degree angle and pump your arms up and down while inhaling for five counts and exhaling for five counts. Repeat for ten breaths.

- **Pilates Roll-Up**

  Begin by lying on your back with your arms extended overhead. Slowly roll up, reaching for your toes, and then roll back down one vertebra at a time. Aim for six to eight repetitions.

- **Pilates Plank**

  Assume a plank position with your hands directly under your shoulders and your body forming a straight line. Hold this position for a challenging yet manageable amount of time, gradually increasing as you build strength.

Exercise 5: Yoga

- **Stress reduction:** Yoga is known for its stress-reducing benefits. High levels of stress can lead to hair loss or exacerbate existing hair conditions, such as alopecia areata or telogen effluvium. By practising yoga regularly, individuals may experience reduced stress levels, which can positively impact hair health.
- **Improved blood circulation:** Certain yoga poses involve stretching and inversions that can improve blood circulation throughout the body, including the scalp. Better blood circulation means increased delivery of oxygen and nutrients to hair follicles, potentially supporting healthier hair growth.
- **Balancing hormones:** Some yoga practices focus on the endocrine system, which plays a role in hormone regulation. Hormonal imbalances can contribute to hair loss, especially in conditions like androgenetic alopecia. Yoga's potential to balance hormones may indirectly benefit hair health.

- **Enhanced relaxation and sleep:** Poor sleep and inadequate relaxation can impact overall health, including hair health. Yoga promotes relaxation and can improve the quality of sleep, which is essential for cell regeneration and overall well-being, potentially benefiting the hair growth cycle.
- **Positivity and mindfulness:** Practising yoga encourages a positive and mindful approach to life. A positive mindset and emotional well-being can impact overall health, leading to a healthier body, including hair.

Child's Pose (Balasana):

- Kneel on the floor with your big toes touching and knees spread wide.
- Sit back on your heels and extend your arms forward, resting your forehead on the mat.
- Hold for several deep breaths, relaxing the body and mind.

Forward Fold (Uttanasana):

- Stand with your feet hip-width apart.
- Exhale and bend forward from the hips, reaching your hands towards the ground or your shins.
- Let your head hang and relax your neck.
- Hold for a few breaths, feeling the stretch along your back and hamstrings.

Seated Forward Bend (Paschimottanasana):

- Sit on the floor with your legs extended in front of you.
- Inhale and lengthen your spine, then exhale as you bend forward from your hips.
- Reach for your feet or ankles or place your hands on your shins, depending on your flexibility.
- Hold the pose for several breaths, feeling the stretch along your back and hamstrings.

Legs Up the Wall (Viparita Karani):

- Lie on your back near a wall and lift your legs up the wall.
- Keep your buttocks close to the wall and let your arms rest by your sides.
- Relax and focus on deep, slow breathing as you stay in this pose for a few minutes.

Corpse Pose (Savasana):

- Lie on your back with your arms at your sides and your palms facing up.
- Close your eyes and let your body completely relax.
- Focus on your breath and stay in this pose for several minutes.

Vegetarian Diet Plan for Healthy Hair

Early morning: 1 glass lukewarm water with 1 tsp of apple cider vinegar and 1 tsp turmeric

Breakfast: 1 glass pineapple nuts green smoothie

Mid-morning: 1 seasonal fruit

Lunch: 1 bowl dal, 1 bowl leafy vegetable, 1 ragi roti, 1 bowl curd, salad and pickle

Evening snack: 1 cup herbal detox tea by Nutracy Lifestyle with 1 'Snack a protein bar' by Nutracy Lifestyle

Dinner: Drumstick soup with quinoa pulav

Non-Vegetarian Diet Plan for Healthy Hair

Early morning: 1 glass warm water with 1 tsp A2-cow ghee

Breakfast:

Option 1: 1 glass green smoothie

Option 2: 1 glass almond oat smoothie

Lunch:

Option 1: Chicken-stuffed mushroom omelette

Option 2: Avocado egg toast

Snacks: 1 glass beauty collagen drink

Dinner:

Option 1: Chicken curry with 1 bowl of quinoa and 1 bowl of mixed salad

Option 2: Grilled fish with 1 bowl of sweet potato tofu salad

GROCERY LIST

Maintaining a healthy diet is crucial for promoting overall well-being, including hair health. Including nutrient-rich foods that support hair growth and scalp health can be beneficial. Here's a grocery list of items that can contribute to healthy hair:

Protein Sources:

- ☐ Eggs
- ☐ Fish (salmon, mackerel, sardines)
- ☐ Lean meats (chicken, turkey)
- ☐ Legumes (lentils, chickpeas, beans)
- ☐ Nuts and seeds (almonds, walnuts, chia seeds)

Fruits and Vegetables (Rich in Vitamins and Antioxidants):

- ☐ Spinach
- ☐ Kale
- ☐ Berries (blueberries, strawberries, raspberries)

- ☐ Sweet potatoes
- ☐ Bell peppers
- ☐ Citrus fruits (oranges, grapefruits)

Whole Grains:

- ☐ Brown rice
- ☐ Quinoa
- ☐ Oats

Healthy Fats:

- ☐ Avocado
- ☐ Olive oil
- ☐ Fatty fish (salmon, trout)
- ☐ Nuts and seeds

Dairy or Dairy Alternatives (Rich in Calcium and Protein):

- ☐ Greek yoghurt
- ☐ Almond milk
- ☐ Soy milk

Biotin-Rich Foods:

- ☐ Eggs
- ☐ Nuts and seeds
- ☐ Sweet potatoes
- ☐ Cauliflower

Iron Sources:

- ☐ Red meat
- ☐ Spinach
- ☐ Lentils
- ☐ Chickpeas

Zinc-Rich Foods:

- ☐ Oysters
- ☐ Pumpkin seeds
- ☐ Chickpeas
- ☐ Spinach

Vitamin C Sources:

- ☐ Citrus fruits
- ☐ Strawberries
- ☐ Kiwi
- ☐ Guava

Omega-3 Fatty Acid Sources:

- ☐ Fatty fish (salmon, mackerel and trout)
- ☐ Flaxseeds
- ☐ Chia seeds
- ☐ Walnuts

Healthy Grocery List

GLUTEN FREE & VEGAN

Long Lasting Items to Stock Up With

Fruit:

- apples
- bananas
- oranges
- avocados
- dried fruit

Vegetables:

- lemons
- carrots
- onions
- garlic
- squash
- spinach
- kale
- peppers
- green beans
- cucumbers
- broccoli
- ginger
- mushrooms
- potatoes

Protein:

- lentils
- soy-based tempeh
- veggie burgers
- spirulina
- nut butters
- tahini
- beyond burgers

Fridge Staples:

- almond milk
- sauerkraut
- vegan mayo
- vegan yogurt
- vegan cheese
- vegan butter
- pesto
- hummus
- salsa
- condiments

Pantry Items:

- chia seeds
- flaxseeds
- nuts
- seeds
- honey
- maple syrup
- cacao nibs
- shredded coconut
- coconut aminos
- Apple Cider Vinegar

Canned Foods/ Non-Perishables:

- tomato sauce
- tomato paste
- beans
- chickpeas
- coconut milk
- apple sauce
- almond milk
- coconut water
- vegetable broth

Pasta & Grains:

- quinoa
- rice
- GF pasta
- GF seeded bread
- GF rolled oats
- GF steel cut oats
- GF granola
- rice cakes
- brown rice wraps

Snacks & Chips:

- popcorn
- roasted seaweed
- goMacro bars
- seeded crackers
- tortilla chips

Freezer:

- pre-chopped veggies
- fruit (blueberries/mixed, etc.)
- cauliflower gnocchi
- Daily Harvest Smoothies & Bowls
- Amy's Kitchen Pre-made Meals

Other:

- water & tea
- GF baking ingredients
- Himalayan salt & black pepper
- olive or avocado oil
- nutritional yeast

The power of infrared lights on your hair

Infrared light therapy for hair is a type of light therapy that uses infrared light to stimulate hair growth and improve the health of the hair follicles. Infrared light falls within the electromagnetic spectrum and has longer wavelengths than visible light, making it capable of penetrating deeper into the tissues.

The concept behind infrared light therapy for hair is similar to other forms of light therapy. When infrared light is applied to the scalp, it is believed to do the following:

- **Enhance blood circulation:** Infrared light is thought to improve blood flow to the scalp, which can increase the supply of oxygen and nutrients to the hair follicles.
- **Activate cellular metabolism:** The light may stimulate cellular activity in the hair follicles, promoting energy production and protein synthesis, which can improve hair follicle health.
- **Reduce inflammation:** Infrared light has anti-inflammatory properties, which can be beneficial for hair follicles that are inflamed or damaged.

Infrared light therapy for hair can be administered through various devices, such as infrared helmets, caps, combs or panels. Treatment sessions typically involve exposing the scalp to infrared light for a specific duration, often a few minutes per session, a few times per week.

As with any hair loss treatment, results may vary from person to person, and individual responses to infrared light therapy can differ. It's essential to consult with a healthcare professional or dermatologist before starting any hair loss treatment, including infrared light therapy. They can assess your specific hair loss condition, determine if infrared light therapy is suitable for you, and provide guidance on the proper use of devices or in-office treatments if available.

Light therapy for hair, also known as low-level laser therapy (LLLT) or photobiomodulation, is a non-invasive treatment that uses low-level lasers or light-emitting diodes (LEDs) to stimulate hair growth and improve the health of the hair follicles. The concept behind this therapy is that specific wavelengths of light can be absorbed by the hair follicles, promoting cellular activity and improving blood flow in the scalp, leading to thicker, healthier hair.

There are different methods of light therapy for hair, including:

- **Laser helmets and caps:** These are devices that resemble regular caps or helmets equipped with low-level lasers or LEDs. Users wear them for a specific duration, typically a few minutes per session, a few times per week.
- **Laser combs:** These handheld devices incorporate low-level lasers or LEDs and are moved over the scalp to target specific areas.
- **Laser panels:** These are larger devices that emit light over a broader area, allowing for more coverage of the scalp during treatment.

The exact mechanisms by which light therapy stimulates hair growth are not entirely understood, but some proposed theories include:

- **Increased blood flow:** Light therapy is thought to improve blood circulation in the scalp, delivering more oxygen and nutrients to the hair follicles.
- **Activation of dormant hair follicles:** Light therapy may awaken hair follicles that have become inactive or dormant, leading to new hair growth.
- **Modulation of cellular activity:** The light may stimulate cellular metabolism and protein synthesis, promoting hair follicle health and hair growth.

DAILY HAIR HEALTH CHECKLIST

[Put a tick before the task when completed.]

- ☐ Today, I had all my essential vitamins in check.
- ☐ Today, my breakfast, lunch and dinner plates were colourful and nourishing.
- ☐ Today, I had 8 glasses of water.
- ☐ Today, I meditated for 15 minutes.
- ☐ Today, I did some form of physical activity.
- ☐ Today, I did not excessively brush my hair and did hair massaging.
- ☐ Today, I meditated before going to sleep and cared for my health.

Daily Haircare:

- ☐ **Gentle brushing:** Use a soft-bristle brush or wide-tooth comb to detangle hair gently, starting from the ends and working your way up.
- ☐ **Avoid over-washing:** Wash your hair every 2–3 days (or as needed) to prevent stripping natural oils from the scalp.
- ☐ **Use a silk or satin pillowcase:** Sleeping on a silk or satin pillowcase can reduce friction and prevent hair breakage.
- ☐ **Stay hydrated:** Drink plenty of water throughout the day to keep your body and scalp hydrated.
- ☐ **Balanced diet:** Consume a nutritious diet rich in vitamins, minerals and protein to support healthy hair growth.

Weekly Haircare:

- ☐ **Deep conditioning treatment:** Apply a deep conditioner or hair mask once a week to nourish and hydrate your hair.
- ☐ **Scalp massage:** Massage your scalp weekly to stimulate blood flow and promote hair growth.
- ☐ **Trimming:** Trim split ends every 6–8 weeks to maintain healthy hair and prevent further damage.

Monthly Haircare:

- ☐ **Clarifying shampoo:** Use a clarifying shampoo once a month to remove product buildup and excess oils.

- ☐ **Hot oil treatment:** Apply a hot oil treatment to your hair once a month for added moisture and shine.

Hair Styling Practices:

- ☐ **Limit heat styling:** Minimize the use of heat styling tools, such as blow dryers, straighteners, and curling irons. Use heat-protectant products when styling.
- ☐ **Avoid tight hairstyles:** Avoid hairstyles that put excessive tension on your hair, such as tight ponytails or braids.
- ☐ **Protect from UV rays:** When exposed to the sun, wear a hat or use hair products containing UV protection to shield your hair from harmful sun rays.

General Tips:

- ☐ **Regular haircuts:** Visit a hairstylist every 6–8 weeks to keep your hair looking fresh and healthy.
- ☐ **Avoid chemical treatments:** Limit the use of harsh chemical treatments like perms, relaxers, and bleach, as they can damage the hair.
- ☐ **Use quality hair products:** Choose haircare products that are suitable for your hair type and free from sulphates and parabens.
- ☐ **Minimize stress:** Manage stress through relaxation techniques like yoga or meditation, as stress can contribute to hair loss.

HAIRCARE GUIDE: CONCLUSION

- In conclusion, a well-balanced and nutrient-rich diet is the foundation for maintaining healthy and vibrant hair. Proper haircare involves ensuring an adequate intake of essential nutrients such as protein, B vitamins, vitamin C, vitamin A, vitamin E, iron and omega-3 fatty acids. These nutrients play vital roles in promoting hair growth, preventing hair loss, and enhancing the overall health and appearance of our hair.
- Including a variety of foods such as nuts, seeds, legumes, meat, fish, fruits, vegetables, whole grains, and dairy products can help provide the necessary nutrients for optimal hair health. Additionally, staying hydrated by drinking plenty of water is essential for supporting hair growth and maintaining scalp health.
- While a nutrient-dense diet is crucial, it's also important to avoid crash diets or extreme restrictions as they can deprive the body of essential nutrients and negatively impact hair health.

- In addition to proper nutrition, other lifestyle factors such as managing stress, getting enough sleep and avoiding excessive heat styling and chemical treatments can also contribute to healthier hair.
- Remember that individual needs may vary, and consulting with healthcare professionals or registered dietitians can provide personalized guidance and recommendations based on specific hair concerns and health conditions.
- By adopting a holistic approach to haircare nutrition and overall wellness, we can ensure that our hair stays strong, shiny, and beautiful for years to come.

BIBLIOGRAPHY

Grymowicz, M., Rudnicka, E., Podfigurna, A., Napierala, P., Smolarczyk, R., Smolarczyk, K., & Meczekalski, B. (2020). Hormonal Effects on Hair Folicles. *International journal of molecular sciences*, 21(15), 5342. https://doi.org/10.3390/ijms21155342

Ho, B. S., Ho, E., Chu, C. W., Ramasamy, S., Bigliardi-Qi, M., de Sessions, P. F., & Bigliardi, P. L. (2019). Microbiome in the hair follicle of androgenetic alopecia patients. *PloS one*, 14(5), e0216330. https://doi.org/10.1371/journal.pone.0216330)

Vitamin D (Bikle, D., & Christakos, S. (2020). New aspects of vitamin D metabolism and action - addressing the skin as source and target. *Nature reviews. Endocrinology*, 16(4), 234–252. https://doi.org/10.1038/s41574-019-0312-5)

IBS and hair loss (Patel, K. V., Farrant, P., Sanderson, J. D., & Irving, P. M. (2013). Hair loss in patients with inflammatory bowel disease. *Inflammatory bowel diseases*, 19(8), 1753–1763. https://doi.org/10.1097/MIB.0b013e31828132de)

Schneier FR. Social anxiety disorder. *BMJ* 2003; 327: 515–6 PubMed Central. https://doi.org/10.1136/bmj.327.7414.515

Trüeb, R. M., Henry, J. P., Davis, M. G., & Schwartz, J. R. (2018). Scalp Condition Impacts Hair Growth and Retention via Oxidative Stress. *International journal of trichology,* 10(6), 262–270. https://doi.org/10.4103/ijt.ijt_57_18

Krajmalnik-Brown, R., Ilhan, Z. E., Kang, D. W., & DiBaise, J. K. (2012). Effects of gut microbes on nutrient absorption and energy regulation. Nutrition in clinical practice : official publication of the American Society for Parenteral and Enteral

Nutrition, 27(2), 201–214. https://doi.org/10.1177/0884533611436116

Jung, D. R., Yoo, H. Y., Kim, M. J., Singh, V., Park, S. H., Jeong, M., Park, B. J., & Shin, J. H. (2022). Comparative analysis of scalp and gut microbiome in androgenetic alopecia: A Korean cross-sectional study. *Frontiers in Microbiology,* 13, 1076242. https://doi.org/10.3389/fmicb.2022.1076242

Sánchez-Pellicer, P., Navarro-Moratalla, L., Núñez-Delegido, E., Agüera-Santos, J., & Navarro-López, V. (2022). How Our Microbiome Influences the Pathogenesis of

Alopecia Areata. Genes, 13(10), 1860. https://doi.org/10.3390/genes13101860

Constantinou, A., Kanti, V., Polak-Witka, K., Blume-Peytavi, U., Spyrou, G. M., & Vogt, A. (2021). The Potential Relevance of the Microbiome to Hair Physiology and Regeneration:

The Emerging Role of Metagenomics. *Biomedicines*, 9(3), 236. https://doi.org/10.3390/biomedicines9030236

Sattur, S. S., & Sattur, I. S. (2021). COVID-19 Infection: Impact on Hair. Indian journal of plastic surgery : official publication of the Association of Plastic Surgeons of India, 54(4), 521–526. https://doi.org/10.1055/s-0041-1740289

Babbu, S. N., & Velusamy, A. (2020). An updated review on hair growth promoting plants. *Journal of Ayurveda and Integrative Medicine*, 11(1), 73–80.

Guo, E. L., & Katta, R. (2017). Diet and hair loss: effects of nutrient deficiency and supplement use. Dermatology Practical & Conceptual, 7(1), 1–10.

Gavazzoni Dias, M. F. R. (2015). Hair cosmetics: an overview. *International Journal of Trichology*, 7(1), 2–15.

Suneetha, W. J., Krishnan, S., & Arun, A. B. (2021). Diet and hair health: an overview. *Journal of Cosmetic Dermatology*, 20(4), 1063-1070.

Beoy, L. A., Woei, W. J., & Hay, Y. K. (2010). Effects of tocotrienol supplementation on hair growth in human volunteers. *Tropical Life Sciences Research*, 21(2), 91–99.

Peker, F., Bali, E. B., & Goker, E. N. (2016). The effects of biotin supplementation on serum and liver tissue biotinidase enzyme activity and alopecia in rats which were administered to valproic acid. Clinical Nutrition Experimental, 6, 13–20.

Staufenbiel, Sabine M., et al. Hair cortisol, stress exposure, and mental health in humans: a systematic review. *Psychoneuroendocrinology* 38.8 (2013): 1220–1235.

Guo, E. L., & Katta, R. (2018). Diet and hair loss: effects of nutrient deficiency and supplement use. *Dermatology Practical & Conceptual,* 9(1), 1–10.

Byrd, A., Belkaid, Y. & Segre, J. The human skin microbiome. *Nat Rev Microbiol* 16, 143–155 (2018). https://doi.org/10.1038/nrmicro.2017.157

Cao, C., Xiao, Z., Wu, Y., & Ge, C. (2020). Diet and Skin Aging-From the Perspective of Food Nutrition. *Nutrients, 12*(3), 870. https://doi.org/10.3390/nu12030870

Elizabeth Street. "Improve Your Skin Just By Changing Your Diet." Elizabeth Street, n.d., https://elizabethstreet.com/improve-your-skin-just-by-changing-your-diet/.

A NOTE OF GRATITUDE

As I close this chapter of my journey, I am overwhelmed with gratitude for each and every one of you who has been a part of bringing this book to life. To my family and my Nutracy Lifestyle team, your unwavering support and encouragement have been the fuel behind every word written. Your love and understanding have been my guiding light, and I am forever grateful for your presence in my life.

I also extend my heartfelt appreciation to Ketki Mungi and Harshita Karle for their invaluable assistance and collaboration. Your contributions have enriched this project and infused it with depth and excellence.

To all the readers who have shown interest in this book, thank you for your curiosity and dedication. It is my sincere hope that this book serves as a beacon of knowledge on your journey to better health and well-being.

With deepest gratitude and warmest regards,

Dr Rohini Patil

ABOUT THE AUTHOR

DR ROHINI PATIL
Doctor (MBBS), DDHN (Health and Education),
DDSEN (Sports and Exercise Nutrition)
Certified in Anti-Aging, Ovarian Disease Management and Weight Management

Dr Rohini Somnath Patil is a highly accomplished and multitalented individual with a remarkable vision and perspective. Armed with several specialized certifications in health and nutrition, she has made significant contributions to the fields of diet and lifestyle modifications. Hailing from Maharashtra, India, she is a distinguished figure in the field of diet and nutrition. She graduated with an MBBS, distinguishing herself as one of the very few MBBS doctors who have ventured into the realm of diet and wellness. Her passion for promoting healthy lifestyles and her commitment to improving people's well-being have made her a leading expert in her field. Over the last ten years, she has ardently researched various aspects of health, including diet, nutrition, fitness, mental well-being and overall lifestyle improvement.

Dr Patil is the founder and CEO of **Nutracy Lifestyle**, a pioneering venture that focuses on diet, fitness and lifestyle modifications with disease/concern-based diet consultations, biohacking fat-loss therapies, DNA-based genetic testing.

She is the founder of **Nutracy Essentials**, promoting her chain of authentic, uniquely crafted health- and-wellness products like herbal teas, energy bars, marine collagen and many more lined-up health supplements and wellness products.

She is the founder of **Nutracy Academy** with listed courses on Skin Glow, Weight Loss, Hormonal Imbalance and many more.

Dr Patil is also the founder of **Nutracy Wellness Community**, which focuses on elevating well-being with an approach of mindful living.

As part of her dedication to spreading awareness and promoting healthy living, Dr Patil conducts regular seminars and workshops. These events offer her clients and audiences valuable insights and practical guidance, illuminating the path towards a fulfilling and healthy lifestyle. She also has a YouTube Channel titled 'Dr Rohini Patil' which deals with diet, nutrition and lifestyle guidance.

The Lifestyle Diet by Dr Rohini Patil—published by HarperCollins *Publishers* India in 2021 and translated into different regional Indian languages: Hindi and Marathi—focuses on reinventing a healthy lifestyle in the modern world.

Through her writing, she aims to inspire and empower people to make informed choices about their health and well-being. She also has a weekly column about health, nutrition and wellness in *Pune Mirror* (*The Times of India*) and *Sakal* newspaper. Since the last two years, Dr Patil has also been hosting a radio show called 'Healthy Lifestyle with Dr Rohini' on Radio 94.3 Tomato in Kolhapur, Maharashtra.

Dr Patil is a renowned TEDx speaker, known for her expertise in health and nutrition.

She has appeared in various media sources like *Hindustan Times, The Times of India,* Global Spa, Your Story, Tata Cliq, *Femina, India Today, Grazia* India, HT Health Shots, Zoom, *Cosmopolitan, The Pioneer, Social Ketchup* magazine, *India Today Home, The Indian Express,* TV9, Only My Health, Pinkvilla, iDiva, iDiva Hindi, *Vogue, The Post* India, *Provoke* magazine, *The New Indian Express,* IANS, ABP News Channel, *Business World, The Tribune,* HT Health Shots Live, Zee Zest, *The Sunday Standard,* Miss Malini, *ELLE, The Lifestyle Journalist* magazine, *Health and Fashion* magazine, Infuser, PEAKLIFE, HerZindagi, Tweak India, *Global Spa* magazine, The Health Site, News18, TheHealthsite, *Print, The Deccan Chronicle, Times Interact* magazine, Zee News, ABP Live, India TV, Zee News, IANS Life, *HT City, GQ India,* Lokmat Times, *Mid-Day.*

In recognition of her outstanding contributions to the domain of nutrition and her impactful presence, Dr Patil has received the FSSAI Eat Right award (as a social media influencer) which is a national-level award from our Honourable (former) Union Health Minister Dr Harsh Vardhan and Honourable (former) Minister of State (Maharashtra) for Health and Family Welfare Mr Ashwini Choubey. The award was presented on the momentous occasion of the first-ever World Food Safety Day, a testament to her commitment to raising awareness and promoting healthy eating habits. She was recently awarded the BW Wellbeing 30 Under 30 Awards 2023, which is a well-known jury award, for being among the top 30 leaders in the Indian wellness industry as recognized by *Business World* magazine.

She has also been awarded the Professional Health 2016 and Indian Health 2018–19 awards.

Dr Patil has been recognized as an official nutritionist on board with National Indian Athletes, including esteemed organizations like GAIL and NYCS. Her involvement in the world of sports nutrition has allowed her to contribute to the performance and well-being of athletes, enhancing their dietary practices for optimal results. Her remarkable entrepreneurship, achievements and leadership have earned her prestigious recognitions.

Dr Patil's remarkable professional capabilities have led her to serve as the head and second-NMO president of the Medical Students Association of India (MSAI), the largest and leading medical students' association in the country.

She also headed the Indian delegation in the USA organized by International Federation of Medical Students Association (IFMSA) and American Medical Students Association (AMSA) general assembly held at Baltimore and Washington, D.C. She was a part of the core organizing committee of MEDIACE (a national-level UG and PG medical students' conference). She has also been a winner at the National Debate in MEDIACE.

She has also been a national-level lawn tennis player. She is a student of Mahesh Bhupati Tennis Academy, Bengaluru.

Furthermore, she is a highly accomplished athlete, having won a gold medal in the National Inter Medical Lawn Tennis Tournament at AIIMS, Delhi, and is a national-level lawn tennis player.

Dr Rohini Patil's journey is a testament to her dedication, passion and relentless pursuit of excellence in the realms of health, nutrition and lifestyle. Her contributions have inspired many, making her a true trailblazer in her field and beyond. Dr Patil's passion, expertise and drive have made her an esteemed figure in the field of diet and nutrition in India. Her contributions to the well-being of individuals and her commitment to advancing the cause of a healthy lifestyle continue to impact lives positively, making her a beacon of inspiration for many seeking to lead healthier and more fulfilling lives.

HarperCollins *Publishers* India

At HarperCollins India, we believe in telling the best stories and finding the widest readership for our books in every format possible. We started publishing in 1992; a great deal has changed since then, but what has remained constant is the passion with which our authors write their books, the love with which readers receive them, and the sheer joy and excitement that we as publishers feel in being a part of the publishing process.

Over the years, we've had the pleasure of publishing some of the finest writing from the subcontinent and around the world, including several award-winning titles and some of the biggest bestsellers in India's publishing history. But nothing has meant more to us than the fact that millions of people have read the books we published, and that somewhere, a book of ours might have made a difference.

As we look to the future, we go back to that one word—a word which has been a driving force for us all these years.

Read.

Harper Collins
4th
HARPER FICTION
HARPER NON-FICTION
HARPER BUSINESS
HarperCollins *Children'sBooks*
HARPER DESIGN
Harper Sport
HARPER PERENNIAL
HARPER VANTAGE
हार्पर हिन्दी